NEW DIRECTIONS IN STUTTERING
Theory and Practice

Publication Number 602
AMERICAN LECTURE SERIES®

A Monograph in
The BANNERSTONE DIVISION *of*
AMERICAN LECTURES IN COMMUNICATION

Edited by
DOMINICK A. BARBARA, M.D., F.A.P.A.
Head of the Speech Department
Karen Horney Clinic
New York, New York

NEW DIRECTIONS IN STUTTERING

Theory and Practice

Compiled and Edited by

DOMINICK A. BARBARA, M.D.

Practicing Psychoanalyst
Associated with the American Institute for Psychoanalysis
Head of the Speech Department
Karen Horney Clinic
New York, New York

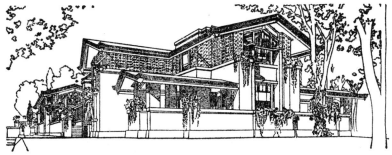

CHARLES C THOMAS • PUBLISHER

Springfield • Illinois • U.S.A.

Published and Distributed Throughout the World by
CHARLES C THOMAS • PUBLISHER
BANNERSTONE HOUSE
301-327 East Lawrence Avenue, Springfield, Illinois, U.S.A.
NATCHEZ PLANTATION HOUSE
735 North Atlantic Boulevard, Fort Lauderdale, Florida, U.S.A.

With THOMAS BOOKS careful attention is given to all details of manufacturing and design. It is the Publisher's desire to present books that are satisfactory as to their physical qualities and artistic possibilities and appropriate for their particular use. THOMAS BOOKS will be true to those laws of quality that assure a good name and good will.

Printed in the United States of America
A-2

CONTRIBUTORS

JANICE P. ALPER, M.A.: *Teaching Fellow in the Department of English and Speech Education, New York University.*

DOMINICK A. BARBARA, M.D.: *Practicing Psychoanalyst associated with the American Institute for Psychoanalysis.*

SMILEY BLANTON, M.D.: *Director of the American Foundation of Religion and Psychiatry.*

OLIVER BLOODSTEIN, PH.D.: *Associate Professor of Speech, Brooklyn College.*

RUTH MILLBURN CLARK, PH.D.: *Professor of Speech, University of Denver.*

EUGENE B. COOPER, ED.D.: *Director of the Adult Therapy Program, Speech and Hearing Clinic, The Pennsylvania State University.*

T. EARLE JOHNSON, PH.D.: *Professor and Head, Department of Speech, University of Alabama.*

EDWIN W. MARTIN, PH.D.: *Associate Professor of Speech, University of Alabama.*

FREDERICK PEMBERTON MURRAY, M.A.: *University Fellow, University of Denver.*

WILLIAM H. PERKINS, PH.D.: *Director of Speech and Hearing Clinic, University of Southern California.*

GEORGE H. SHAMES, PH.D.: *Professor of Speech and Psychology, University of Pittsburgh.*

CARL E. SHERRICK, JR., PH.D.: *Research Psychologist, Princeton University.*

LOUISE M. WARD, M.A.: *Assistant Professor of Speech, University of Alabama.*

PAULETTE M. ZISK, M.A.: *Lecturer in Speech, Brooklyn College.*

In memory of
DOCTOR C. S. BLUEMEL
and his contribution to the
understanding of stuttering

CONTENTS

NEW DIRECTIONS IN STUTTERING

Theory and Practice

1

Stuttering

Smiley Blanton, M.D.

Speech is the index of the mind, says Seneca; not only the index, but the very medium through which the mind is formed and developed. That is why courses in speech should occupy an important position in the curriculum of every school and college. The person who graduates from school or college unable to speak his mother tongue clearly, rhythmically, and idiomatically both in public and private, is not educated. It, of course, follows that no child should leave school with a defect of speech if it is possible to remedy it. Even such slight defects as a mild slurring of the speech or a lisp should receive treatment. Especially should that serious speech disorder, stuttering, receive the attention of teachers everywhere. For stuttering not only causes a blocking or hesitation in the outward speech, but disturbs the emotions so that clear thinking is often impossible.

Stuttering may show itself as a complete blocking of the speech or a repetition of initial sounds or any imaginable combination of these two symptoms. There are many cases in which there is never any outward sign of spasms of the speech organs, but a constant fear that stuttering will occur; many words are dreaded, and there is a constant substitution of one word for another. Such a case was that of an engineer who had no sign whatever of a stutter, but felt that there were hundreds of words that he could not say. His high school and college years had been marked by suffering; every class was an ordeal.

With persons who do stutter, the symptoms vary a great deal. A very brilliant college student, a junior in college at seventeen, never stutters when he works in his father's store, nor when with his companions, but only in his chemistry classes. Chemistry is his major in college; he likes the subject and is doing well in it; and yet it is in this subject that he stutters. A girl of sixteen stutters only in one class in school where there is a most unpleasant teacher. A business man stutters only over the telephone.

There is no dividing line between the frank stutterer who shows all the typical symptoms of blocking and hesitation and the person who is nervous, embarrassed, and timid when the social situation calls for speech. There are many such persons who find it difficult to recite. They often cover up their embarrassment by a refusal to speak. Such refusal is not infrequently interpreted by the teacher as sullenness or obstinacy. An example is that of a man of thirty years of age who lived in the country until he finished his junior year in high school, when the family moved to town and the boy entered a large city high school. Here he was embarrassed and overawed; he felt sensitive about his clothes and his ignorance of city ways; he found it difficult to recite. As he said, "I just could not make myself talk. The words would not come. My tongue seemed to cleave to the roof of my mouth." And yet there were no typical signs of stuttering. His teachers thought him a sullen stupid fellow, and the boy dropped out of school in the middle of his senior year. His life ambition to go to college was made impossible by a lack of understanding on the part of his teachers.

From 5 to 10 per cent of students in high school and college suffer such feelings of inadequacy and embarrassment in reciting that they need the teachers' sympathetic understanding and help. Although these individuals do not show the usual signs of spasms of the speech organs, they suffer from the same inhibition of speech as the stutterer does.

Speech is a medium of group social adjustment. When the creatures began to live in groups, the vocal cords were developed so that they could warn one another of dangers—could attract one another—could express their rage and anger and so escape being overwhelmed or destroyed. Human speech was evolved out of these first primitive cries and calls and songs. Human speech remains primarily a means of expressing the emotions, the chief way in which the child, just emerging from helpless infancy, adjusts itself to the group in an adult way. Stuttering is a symptom of an inability to adjust to the group. It is caused by a fear, a timidity, or a negative (hate) attitude toward the group. With his conscious mind, the child wishes to talk, but with the unconscious mind there is an inhibition against speech. Stuttering is the result. It is hard to believe that there could be such a double motive in stuttering, but analysis of the unconscious mind of the stutterer has proved that such is the case.

The region made up of the mouth, tongue, lips, and throat is highly charged with emotion. Through suckling the infant receives nourishment, and by this act there is produced perhaps the first pleasurable excitement in the life of the infant. For a time the sensations from the oral organs play a predominant part in the development of the emotional life. The oral organs are not only used for the taking of nourishment, but are also connected with the love life. Among the erogenous zones of the body— that is, areas capable of stimulating the sex feelings—is the mouth. The first stage of love life is the oral-erotic stage, in which the child uses the mouth not only to get nourishment, but also to get sexual pleasure—sexual pleasure not in the adult sense, but of a pre-genital, infantile type. The libido, which is the energy derived from the drive of the love impulse, is first largely centered in the mouth. The child gets pleasure by putting not only his thumb or his toe into his mouth, but also almost everything that he can get his hands on. Sounds, too, are made partly because of the pleasure they give through the stimulation of the vocal organs.

This oral-erotic stage, in which the oral organs are highly charged with libido, is in the normal child but a passing phase, although in all cases the mouth remains a very marked erogenous zone. But in some cases the child remains fixed in this oral-erotic stage. The oral organs are overcharged with emotion; the emotional life in some of its aspects remains infantile. Especially in the stutterer does the libido, the love energy, remain fixed upon the individual. He remains in the narcissistic stage, timid and self-centered. It is this narcissism, which gives rise to timidity and self-consciousness, that makes it so difficult for the stutterer to meet the group—to talk to people. Very often such cases are morbidly interested in their own reactions and not infrequently develop an anxiety about their health. They are, as we say, in love with their own bodies; their stomachs, heads, sinuses, or bowels are cherished like a beloved baby.

An example will make things clearer. A boy of eighteen, in perfect health, weighing one hundred and eighty pounds and six feet tall, has a slight stutter. An only child, the attention he received fixed his libido on himself. He worried about every pimple that came on his skin. The boys teased him because he had a dozen ointments for his face. One day he limped into my office with a sprained ankle. He wondered if he needed a plaster cast. It was a very superficial strain, so I bandaged it and told him to walk about moderately on the foot. He came back next day with two sticks. He had put so much liniment on the foot that he had a small blister on it. He wanted me to put an elaborate dressing on the small blister. "It's of no importance," I said. "But," said he, "President Coolidge's son died after a small blister on his heel. How do you know that I may not get such an infection?" And he went about on crutches for two weeks.

Another case was that of a man of thirty with two children. He had a silent stutter—no outward symptoms, but a constant substitution of words. His chief worry was his stomach and bowels. He had rumblings after eating, and could eat only certain things; for example, he could not eat raw apples or tomatoes, or fish and milk together. Once, when he was talking about his little boy who was ill, I said, "I can't tell whether you are talking about your baby boy or your baby stomach. Your anxiety and interest in both are the same." Both of these stutterers were very narcissistic. But the latter case was not so much an oralerotic as an anal-erotic. This type is marked by a holding back—a refusal to talk, to spend money, or, in the case of children, to share their belongings.

Perhaps the case of a child of two and a half who began to

stutter at the age of two will be of interest. She was very negative. This means that there was a thwarting of love. Such thwarting occurs most often because the parents do not love the child enough, or because the training is too rigid. Love thwarted changes to hate, and the hate in this case was shown by a resistance to authority. She would not talk unless forced to do so in order to get something she wanted and then she stuttered, blocking on words for several seconds, but at the same time that she began to stutter, she began to refuse to move her bowels. The nurse, mother, and even the father struggled with her sometimes for more than an hour in order to get results. In this case there was no left-handedness, no abnormality of speech, muscle, or nervous system. It was a pure case of oral-anal-erotic stuttering. And the treatment consisted of putting her in another home for two months, retraining the emotions, and freeing the libido.

The physical symptoms of stuttering are explained by the fact that speech is made up of muscle movements that have a more primitive function. Breathing movements, chewing movements, suckling movements, coughing and vomiting movements are all coordinated through the speech area into the unified movements of speech. When there is an emotional blocking of the control of the higher brain centers over these lower brain centers, each lower brain center tends to act independently. But it is the early fixations that determine whether the stuttering shall consist of a repetition of sounds, or a vomitlike blocking, or a suckling movement.

The psychological causes that lie back of stuttering—the fixation of the libido at the oral- or anal-erotic stage and at the narcissistic stage, making the stutterer so sensitive to the attitude of others that he is often unable to speak normally—these factors have been well established. But it may be asked why do these fixations occur—fixations involving primarily the speech? In order to answer this question, there must be a consideration of the environment of the stutterer, his home conditions, his relations to his family, and the subtle pressures that occur at this formative period.

Stuttering is one of the most difficult problems we have to deal with. It is very hard to understand why a person can speak a word or phrase perfectly in certain situations and in other circumstances almost exactly similar he is unable to speak.

Many years ago I had a patient who was a successful actor. When he was playing a part he never stuttered at all—probably because he was playing a role different from himself. But when he was not playing a part in a play, he stuttered very badly.

I know of several cases of people who only stutter when talking on the telephone. This is understandable, because it is harder to talk to a person on the telephone than face to face.

In my nursery school at Vassar I found that about 10 per cent of the children from two to four stuttered from time to time but the percentage of adult stutterers, as revealed by many surveys, is 2 to 3 per cent. Therefore, it would seem that many children who have an initial stutter when very young overcome it as they grow into adult speech.

I do not feel that there is a clear-cut dividing line between a person with a continual stutter, in which he blocks or repeats words, and the nervous, inhibited, embarrassed individual who finds it difficult to speak at times.

One patient I had was often unable to speak. There was no stutter—the patient would merely say, "I can't talk." I found there was something in his mind which prevented him from speaking, and yet there were no symptoms of stuttering. In my teaching I found a good many such cases of students who were so timid they were unable to recite in class. Unless a teacher recognizes these difficulties, the patient may be considered merely sullen inattentive and not interested in the subject.

In order to understand the symptoms of stuttering it is necessary to learn why people speak. Speech is the one thing that separates man from the lower animals—such as the great apes. This capacity for symbolic communication is a miraculous thing as you see it develop in a young child. I saw a baby the other day, twelve months old, whose mother was feeding her cottage cheese, saying "cheese" with each bite. The baby responded with "cheese" each time her mother said it.

Last summer as I was leaving my house in the morning with two newspapers under my arm, I saw a young child just three years old. As I passed him, he said to his mother "two newspapers". Not only was he keen enough to see there were two newspapers, but he knew the word "two" and the word "newspaper."

I saw another child in the subway and heard him say to his mother, "At least you could have considered it." When you analyze this complex idea expressed in these complex words, one is really amazed at the capacity of children to learn this symbolic communication.

We often lose sight of the wonder, the awe and the mystery of life and one of these great mysteries of life is the capacity of the child to talk. Children speak much better and more quickly if the parents talk to them a great deal. For instance, when dressing a child you can mention the socks, the shoes, etc.; when feeding the child, mention milk, water, butter, bread, etc. If these things are mentioned often enough, the child will develop a much larger vocabulary, speak more quickly and have much less fear of speech. I think it is doubtful if a child so trained will have a stutter.

There are three reasons why we talk. *First,* in order to express emotions. The pitch, quality, volume and rhythm, emphasis, as well as words and gestures express our feelings. These are the most important factors of speech because people rarely listen primarily to what you say, but the way you say it. I think we may quote St. Paul, in the 13th Chapter of Corinthians, "Though I have all faith, so that I could move mountains, and have not charity (love) . . . it profiteth me nothing." So unless you have freed the conscious as well as the unconscious mind of fear, envy and resentment, whatever you say—no matter what the words—will not be effective. People won't like you. Animals and birds have songs, cries, calls, grunts which mean danger, food, warning to flee—but this is not speech. I read recently that a man is in the process of trying to teach a dolphin to talk. Dolphins are very intelligent, but I doubt if he meets with success. Of course parrots speak, but they are mocking birds and merely repeat what is said to them. They never initiate speech.

The *second* function of speech, to repeat, is to adjust us to other people. We are group-living animals and the life of the young animal depends on being with a group and being accepted by the group. A large part of the child's education is based on the speech of the people around him. There are only two ways we can really come close to another person—to talk and to touch him. If you want to be really near to another person you talk to him and touch him at the same time. Everyone knows that when you tell a child a story or read to him, he likes to be held and petted at the same time.

The *third* function of speech—very important, although less so than the others, is to express ideas. But, as I said before, these ideas which we try to express in speech depend to a large extent on the emotional attitudes of the one who is expressing the ideas.

Stuttering, in my opinion, is not a speech defect, because if it were, the person would have the same defect at all times. It is a symptom expressing fear of a group and represents a mal-adjustment of the individual to those around him. The constitutional factors which cause stuttering have long been sought and Dr. Orton maintained that stuttering was caused by conflict between the two hemispheres of the brain. We know that the speech area in the brain is opposite to the preferential hand. We have examples of people who are right-handed and are injured on the left side of the brain and are unable to talk. On the other hand a left-handed person injured on the right side of the brain also loses the capacity to talk. Dr. Orton felt that the speech area was not firmly developed in one hemisphere and there was a tendency to have a speech area in both hemispheres and there was conflict between them—which caused stuttering.

Dr. Travis followed Dr. Orton's teachings for many years, but finally gave up this theory and there are very few now who believe in it.

Dr. Freud, with whom I worked for more than a year, said to me that he felt there were constitutional factors in stuttering and, except in rare cases, psychoanalysis alone was not sufficient to effect a cure. Just what these constitutional factors are, no one has been able to determine so far.

I think the physical symptoms of stuttering can be explained by the development of the nervous system, as the infant develops into a mature individual. At first the infant makes many sounds.

I have seen it stated that there are about 600 speech sounds in the various languages. Everyone knows how the baby yells, grunts, hisses, and makes scores of sounds that are not used in civilized speech. There are about 56 sounds in the English language. The infant has to eliminate a great many of the primitive sounds he uses and confine himself to these 56 sounds.

Strangely enough there are no speech organs—since each organ used in speech is used primarily for something else.

(1)   As soon as a child is born he can breathe and cough.

(2)   He can sneeze.

(3)   He can suckle.

(4)   He can swallow.

(5)   He can move his tongue around in various positions, which he has to do in speech.

(6)   He can vomit.

All of these things he can do at birth.

His vocal cords are used to make sounds at first. He yells, calls and apparently just exercises his lungs and vocal cords. When he reaches the age of ten or twelve months, the speech area opposite the preferential hand begins to develop in the cortex of the brain and gradually this speech area takes over these primitive muscle patterns and uses them as far as necessary in order to make the speech sounds.

In stuttering it seems to me that the emotional factors of fear and resentment block off the use of the primitive muscles in the speech area and the stutterer regresses back to the primitive life movements. In other words, the stutterer will make sounds as though he were vomiting, suckling, swallowing, sneezing, coughing or chewing.

If you study the symptoms of stuttering, you can often detect just which one of these primitive life movements have been blocking the speech.

One factor in stuttering is that some children seem to reject speech. They do not begin to talk until they are two or three years of age, even though they have normal or superior intelligence. This block of the development of speech is due in my experience to the fact that the parents do not talk enough to the child; the child does not receive enough love to make him want to respond;

or he receives so much love that he does not find it necessary to talk. I have seen many cases in which there are two children in the family—one three and one half years old and the other two years—where the older child did all the talking, answering every question addressed to the younger child so that he did not learn to talk until he was almost four years old.

I remember the case of a beautiful child, very intelligent, about three years of age, who had four grandparents, her own parents and a nurse to look after her. She simply did not talk. She pointed to anything she wanted. The old nurse who looked after her was a woman of wisdom. She said to me one day, "You know this child is so rich she doesn't have to talk." Finally they refused to give her things unless she asked for them and she began to use words that she knew perfectly well to ask for what she wanted.

The treatment of stuttering comprises physical hygiene, mental hygiene, and speech training.

The physical-hygiene treatment need only be mentioned. It includes good food, exercise, plenty of sleep, and the remedying of physical abnormalities. Avoid having the tonsils and adenoids removed in order to cure stuttering. If they are diseased, have them out by all means. Do not have the frenum of the tongue cut to cure stuttering. All of these operations, including circumcision, are frequently performed to cure stuttering, the idea being that there is some peripheral irritation or defect that causes the condition. The strain of sitting still in school for long hours should be lessened by allowing the child to move and talk occasionally.

Under the term mental hygiene, we include environmental changes in the home and school. The home discipline must be neither too harsh and nagging nor too tender. Rivalry and jealousy of brothers and sisters should be modified or eliminated as far as possible. In short, the application of the best principles of child guidance should be put into practice in the home. We wish to point out most emphatically that teachers working with stuttering children should have their schedules so arranged that they can see the parents from time to time and go into the home occasionally. Without this consultation with the parents and home visiting, only very limited results can be obtained.

In the school room the stutterer should be treated as far as possible like the other children, but the teacher should always keep before her mind the emotional difficulties from which the child suffers. The negative child should not be allowed to cause a feeling of irritation or anger in the teacher. The sullen child may be only timid. Let the stuttering child talk if he wishes to, recite if he can, but do not ask sharp, peremptory questions, and avoid asking the child to speak more slowly or to repeat, and do not anticipate his word when he blocks. If the child is allowed to speak at all, ignore the speech symptoms.

Will the stuttering child cause other children to imitate him? No. Cases caused by imitation are so rare as to be negligible. We think that the great majority of teachers of speech correction will bear us out in this statement.

Under mental hygiene we include also psychotherapy, suggestion, persuasion, and mental analysis, psychoanalysis being a special type of mental analysis.

Now it is difficult to discuss the methods of psychotherapy apart from speech training. Allow me, then, to discuss psychotherapy and speech training together. Speech treatment, as used by the various teachers, consists of:

1. Phonetic training - teaching the stutterer how to make the various consonant and vowel sounds and practice on difficult sounds, syllables and words, and word combinations.
2. Vocal training, which consists of practice on vowel sounds on the various pitches, training in rhythm, pitch volume, and quality.
3. Practice in speech, through such games as playing store or debating or making formal or informal talks.
4. Dramatic work.

As to phonetic training, we believe that it is unwise and makes the stutterer more self-conscious. There may be rare cases of stuttering that need this treatment, cases caused by some organic injury to the brain such as occurs in encephalitis or after birth injuries. But for the average stutterer who can speak smoothly when alone or when not embarrassed, phonetic drill is, we believe, really harmful. In the case of stutterers who have slurring as well as lisping speech, phonetic training may be given, but only after the stuttering has been remedied through psychotherapy and general speech training.

It is true that the stutterer may need training in speech skill. Certainly some cases do. But this cannot be acquired through a conscious manipulation of the speech organs. You cannot learn to control speech organs as you learn to control an arm or a leg. Speech is too automatic for that.

What, then, of breathing exercises? Is not the breathing disturbed in stuttering? Yes, the breathing is disturbed, but this is caused by the emotion that causes the stuttering. Practice in breathing may give the stutterer some relaxation, but if such exercises lead him to think that his stuttering is caused by defective breathing and take his attention from the psychological factors, they will do more harm than good. So often have I heard stutterers say, "My trouble is that my breathing is irregular — that is why I stutter." In such cases it is impossible to get them to consider the psychological factors.

Vocal exercises, such as are used to improve the voice of non-stutterers in any good class of voice training, may be employed, but the stutterer should not be told that they are given to cure his stuttering; only that it is well to improve his voice — its volume, rhythm, pitch, quality.

Dramatic work is especially helpful. Here the stutterer gets out of himself, takes another character, loses for a time his self-centeredness, gains poise and relaxation and a sense of freedom. We find this work our chief mainstay in our speech work for stutters. With small children, pageants as well as plays can be used. The older children and adults make their own costumes and often the scenery. Many opportunities for speech occur in this work. And when the play is given, an audience is invited, so that the players may have the stimulus of speaking before a sympathetic group. Much depends on the attitude of the teacher and the atmosphere created. This is true of all speech work. Psychotherapy is inextricably mixed with all speech work.

There are many exercises that may be given in the beginning in order to instill confidence in the stutterer. Dr. Charles S. Bluemel, in his book, *Mental Aspects of Stammering,* has a well-worked-out program of speech and vocal training for stutterers. In one respect, however, I should disagree with him: I should never ask the stutterer to stop because he was stuttering. During the training period, I say to the stutterer, "Don't bother about your speech. Stuttering is no sin, and you need not feel guilty when you relapse, nor must you gauge your progress solely on your speech improvement, but on your general adjustment as well." In fact, in some cases, I find Professor Dunlap's method of asking the stutterer to try to stutter all he can a helpful device. This is a sort of negative suggestion that may help in selected cases. But we should like to say emphatically that we do not think it wise ever to ask the stutterer to speak more slowly, to repeat his sentences, or to take thought as to how his vocal organs are working.

Relaxation exercises are very helpful. Perhaps the best method of relaxation is that worked out by Dr. Jacobson of Chicago. His book, *Progressive Relaxation; A Physiological and Clinical Investigation of Muscular States and Their Significance in Psychology and Medical Practice,* is very helpful.

There are some excellent devices for gaining the confidence of the stutterer and creating in him courage and hope. In difficult cases, the teacher can read with the stutterer; later she can whisper while the stutterer talks; and still later, she can merely move her lips while the stutterer speaks. Asking the stutterer to whisper and other such devices are helpful.

But all these exercises, as well as much of the vocal work, involves persuasion and suggestion. Persuasion is sometimes defined as influencing a person to do something or believe something by an appeal to his reason. This is only partly true. Persuasion largely involves an emotional element. Suggestion is entirely a matter of the emotions. When you read with the stutterer, you are playing the part of mother to him. It is the same as when you feel the baby. And many of the things that are done to help stutterers are effective, not because they have any value in themselves, but solely because of their emotional appeal.

A word as to this emotional appeal. We all want to have other people love us, using the term love in the psychoanalytical sense. In ordinary words, we may say that we wish people to like us.

There are some people, of course, who are negative and who wish people to dislike them or hate them. A child of this type is most difficult to help. The stuttering child is usually eager for attention — that is, for love. Usually he needs to receive attention and affectionate regard. Now it is this attention and regard which the stutterer receives that often is the chief cause of a change in his attitude and a modification of his emotional conflicts. Speaking psychoanalytically, it is this transfer of the emotions on the part of the stutterer that gets the results. If the teacher has the capacity for gaining this transfer, results may be obtained by any method, no matter how absurd or unreasonable.

Results obtained by this transfer method, however, usually do not last. Only a very few such cases remain cured of their defect. It is quite all right to make use of this transfer to help the stutterer understand himself and his problems, to help him face his difficulties. But, in the end, the transfer must be broken. While retaining a regard for the teacher, the stutterer must be freed of his dependence and no longer expect the teacher to play the part of a tender mother and father.

We see, then, that stuttering is a difficult combination of organic and constitutional and functional factors that requires speech training, such as may be used for the training of the speech and voice of non-stutterers, and that requires also a definite knowledge of mental hygiene in order that hampering emotional fixations may be resolved. These emotional problems cannot be adequately treated by good will and a kind heart and inspirational talks. We believe that an adequate treatment of stuttering must combine physical hygiene, mental hygiene, and speech training in a unified and well-rounded manner.

2

Stuttering: Some Common
Denominators

William H. Perkins, Ph.D.

The search for common denominators in the problem of stuttering has not been fruitful. The only commonality that seems to distinguish with reasonable certainty the person who stutters from the one who does not is the fact of stuttering; and agreement on identifying characteristics of this act is far from complete (Wingate, 1962). Evidence to support psychological or personality differences in the stutterer himself or in his background is, at best, only suggestive (Goodstein, 1958 - Sheehan, 1958). The idea persists that a distinguishing organic variant operates, but conclusive findings to support this possibility have not yet been established. The picture of the person who stutters is sufficiently confused by the contradictory research findings to lead St. Onge (1963) to speculate that a single syndrome of stuttering may not exist; that it may, in fact, be a triple syndrome phenomenon in which stuttering is manifested in one group because of an organic predisposition, in another because of psychogenic factors which produce this symptom, and in another because of a phobic reaction to speech hesitancy.

Nature of the Evidence

Although research evidence does not support the concept of a core problem basic to stutterers, clinical evidence is strongly

17

suggestive that male stutterers, at least, experience the same conflict in relation to the act of stuttering. This impression is based on over 4,000 hours of psychotherapy and counseling with fifty-two stutterers with whom the author has worked during the last ten years. The stutterers themselves have provided the instruction for the formulation of the author's concepts of the conflict. They had to be persistent in their efforts to make him understand how they felt, for he was a slow pupil. Six years of listening, puzzlement, and frustration preceded the development of these ideas in what is essentially their present form. They have been tested clinically during the last four years with twenty one stutterers each of whom has been in therapy from twelve to 200 sessions. All but one have been males, of whom fifteen have been adults.

With each of these individuals, support for the idea of a common conflict was found in several respects. First, stuttering coincided with the periods during which the conflict was active. Second, as it was resolved, the acts of stuttering and concern about blocking diminished without exception, and all but disappeared in at least twelve cases. Third, the interpretations based on these concepts of the conflict were usually validated by the stutterers' recognition that they did experience the feelings that were described.

The clinical observations that support these formulations are, of course, subject to serious limitations. They have all been made by one observer who has, despite his best efforts, doubtless been biased by his theoretical position. In other words, he may have structured clinical situations in which he produced the evidence he wished to observe. It is possible, too, that selective factors have operated to limit the case load with which he worked to a homogeneous group all of whom exhibited the same conflict. Another limitation is the nature of the evidence itself. Much of it is unverified subjective report of feelings, and much of it is report of behavior outside of the therapy setting and accordingly was not directly observed. Nonetheless, the similarity of events reported, subjective experiences described, and metaphorical allusions was sufficiently striking to suggest commonality.

Although these limitations preclude acceptance of the idea of a common conflict on the basis of clinical impressions, such impressions do have a distinct value. They are formulated at a holistic level which allows account to be taken of highly complex behavior which admits to the dynamically shifting influence of un-limited variables. Such conceptualizations are designed as attempts to encompass the full pattern of existence that makes human experience unique (Teilhard de Chardin, 1961). The reductionistic fallacy of trying to explain a complexly organized system by an analysis of its components at a more readily measured molecular level has been avoided specifically. The result appears to be re-warding in that the hypotheses developed about the male stutterer's conflict have provided sufficient predictive power in the clinical situation to warrant closer, more rigorous experimental investigation.

Because holistic concepts can allow for so many alternative explanations as to vitiate a critical test of their validity, the theory of the conflict presented in this chapter has been developed in the form of hypotheses. Even as hypotheses, the ideas do not readily admit to observable operational specification. Still, with ingenuity, predictions of behavioral manifestations can be made which, if supported, will not prove the theory, but if not supported, will defeat it — and this in the final analysis is the measure of a scientific formulation.

The hypotheses developed here have to do with conflict as the stutterer experiences it. The extent to which these hypotheses can be generalized is uncertain. The clinical evidence is predominantly from adult males, but it has appeared to be the same in few females with whom the author has worked. Whether the conflict is experienced similarly when the stuttering stems from organic or from neurotic or from speech-phobic bases, if such distinctions are ever determined to be valid, is problematic. None of the stutterers observed had known organic disability, all were speechphobic at the outset of therapy, and as a group they ranged from minimal to considerable degrees of neuroticism.

Common Dimensions

The suspicion is that the conflict as experienced by stutterers is essentially the same in all cases. This suspicion is strengthened by recognition that the hypothesized commonality among stutterers is far from being unique just to this group. That is to say, the stutterer appears to handle the common conflict by blocking, whereas many, if not most, non-stutterers deal with the same feelings with a variety of other devices. Perhaps this explains why attempts to differentiate stutterers from non-stutterers have been so unproductive. In a sense, the stutterer seems to be struggling with the issue that Hayakawa (1962) states succinctly: "The fundamental motive of human behavior is not self-preservation, but preservation of the symbolic self." If this is the concern that the stutterer handles by blocking, then it is universal; there would be no reason to expect it to differentiate one group from another. A critical question, then, which must be considered is why does the stutterer stutter rather than resolve his conflict in some other manner?

The following discussion of these issues has been organized around three major hypotheses and their corollaries. All of these formulations are so interrelated as to make their organization rather arbitrary. In a sense they are all descriptions of various facets of the same experience, so categorizing and considering them as separate hypotheses violates their unity. It does serve the necessary purpose, though, of stating these various manifestations in sufficiently explicit terms that, hopefully, the concepts can be studied operationally.

Hypothesis I

The overriding concern which seems to be the basic condition for eliciting stuttering is a feeling of loss of impact value. We have all doubtless experienced this feeling in our lives. It may have occurred in a discussion in which we were unable to get a word in edgeways, and if we did, our ideas did not elicit a reaction from the group; the conversation seemed to flow over us and around us, and, try as we might, we were unable to make an effective contribution to it. Or, this valueless feeling may have occurred for us in countless other situations, but in any of them it is as if we had made no impact on others with our presence. It is a painfully frustrating condition from which escape is not easy. If you express your resentment about feeling ignored, then you run the risk of increasing your plight by making a fool of yourself. This is the condition in which the stutterer seems to feel trapped when he blocks. Accordingly, we will formulate the following major hypothesis: *The stutterer experiences at a low level of awareness the feeling that his impact value as a person jeopardized in those situations in which he stutters.*

Corollary Hypothesis I-1

A corollary of Hypothesis I is that *speech is overvalued as a powerful tool with which to effect personal impact.* Stutterers seem to value speech more as a powerful means of exerting influence than as a means of communicating ideas. This results, paradoxically, in addiction to speech. Although stutterers are reported to enjoy speaking less than non-stutterers (Trotter and Bergman, 1957), and although they do obviously communicate ideas, often effectively, they nevertheless seem to be addicted to speaking whether or not they have anything of importance to say. Such remarks from severe stutterers as, "Once I start talking I just can't stop," or "I love words. They're the most powerful, beautiful things I know," attest to the overvaluation of the power of speech. This may account wholly or in part for the selection of speech as the avenue of self-assertion to block automatically; perhaps none other compares with it for making a forcible impact.

Corollary Hypothesis I-2

Another corollary of Hypothesis I is: *the stutterer devalues his actual achievements as a basis for valuing himself.* He seems to feel that what he has accomplished, much as it may be, does not really prove his merit because it really is a shame, a falsification of his true ability; if people really knew him they would see that he had no worth. He feels that his achievements are a result of careful planning and strategy designed to obscure what he fears would otherwise be exposed as a condition of valuelessness. He cannot trust himself to live each moment spontaneously as it comes, so, typically, he crosses his bridges before reaching them. Milisen[1] has been heard on occasion to describe this plight of the stutterer in vivid terms. He has said, in essence, that the difference between the way a non-stutterer and a stutterer approach speech

---

[1]Personal communication with Robert Milisen.

is the same as the difference between the way a farmer crosses a cow pasture in the daytime and at night.

A quiet subdued thirty-year-old longshoreman offers a good example of how valueless outstanding performance can be for a stutterer's appraisal of himself. This man started therapy with a fairly severe problem of stuttering about which he complained bitterly and on which he blamed everything. At the same time, he was working for a college degree. He had received excellent grades and had spent endless hours worrying and studying for his courses. As his stuttering began to disappear, he became openly belligerent, particularly toward those teachers and students who complimented him on his grades. In effect, he shifted his attitude toward speech to his school work. He no longer stuttered nor was concerned about speaking, instead he became increasingly fearful that he would fail in his last semester before graduation, especially in those subjects in which he had done well. When confronted with the excellence of his earlier work, he discounted it as not proving anything because he always performed his achievements secretly. By maintaining anonymity no one would expect anything of him or know about him in the event that he did fail. He distrusted the value of his past performance so much that he said, "I don't dare give up worrying and stewing about these exams, even though I know they're easy and I know the material, because if I went in and just did the best I could I know it wouldn't be enough. I just can't run the risk of finding out for sure that everything I've done is really a big fake."

Disproof of this hypothesis would seem to be found in those stutterers who have made significant contributions and whose speech has improved as their reputations have grown. On the other hand, this may offer confirmation, if this improvement has resulted from the acclaim they have received. The stutterers reported here were heavily dependent on and vulnerable to the attitudes of their listeners; so much so, in fact, that the severity of their stuttering appeared to vary as a function of the importance of their topic as judged by their listeners. They seemed to feel that their own opinions carried so little weight that they had to "second-guess" their audience for significant topics. It was as if they borrowed personal impact by speaking on subjects others considered to be weighty. Stuttering decreased as authorative judgment of significance of the topic increased.

Hypothesis II

The second major hypothesis is: *the act of stuttering reduces anxiety evoked by loss of impact more than it elicits anxiety about the consequences of stuttering.* Introspective reports from adults who stutter tend to confirm what common sense tells us about stuttering—that it is a tension-producing act to be dreaded and avoided. Bloodstein (1960), however, has described this emotional reaction to stuttering as being typical only of the fourth, and final, phase of its development. Moreover, of course, common sense can be misleading; it has been described as "that sense which tells us that the world is flat." The clinical evidence on which this report is based supports strongly the concept that stuttering automatically provides protection against awareness of the painful frustration associated with the feeling of personal devaluation. This is not to deny that the act of stuttering itself is frustrating, but rather to point up why it persists despite this frustration.

Invariably, for those reported here, the stuttering and its consequences were considered the major problem at the outset of treatment. Those who progressed to the point of no longer stuttering or at least no longer considering themselves as stutterers, even though they still blocked occasionally, all made the same change in their point of concern. Some gradually and some abruptly recognized that the problem they faced when they were able to look beyond the stuttering was "preservation of the symbolic self," to use Hayakawa's phrase. This recognition was accompanied by felt-anxiety far in excess of any they had reported when preoccupied with stuttering as their problem.

The most dramatic illustration of what was consistently evident in varying degrees among those who experienced therapeutic change was a twenty-two year old architect who was able to average only fifty to 200 words per hour in the first months of therapy. When he arrived for the session following one in which he had been confronted with the probable defensive value of his stuttering, he was hardly recognizable. He was haggard and unshaven, he looked as if he had not slept, or, if he had it had been in his clothes, but the most startling difference was that he was fluent. He reported that he had been unable to stutter since awakening the morning after our last session. He said he felt raw and exposed, as if he were "walking naked through Times Square." He also said, "I would give anything to get my stuttering back so I could hide behind its protection." He was unable to stutter again and he spent a miserable month adjusting to his exposed condition. His behavior following this period was as different as his speech. Where he had been shy and retiring, he was now overly aggressive; where he had never dated a girl in his life, he was now a veritable Lothario complete with Thunderbird. That significant changes in his life occurred is unquestionable, that they were therapeutic is another matter. Fortunately, he found a wife within the year, settled down to a fairly stable life, and had no further speech trouble until his wife became pregnant four years later, at which time he returned for additional help with a mild recurrence of stuttering.

COROLLARY HYPOTHESIS II-1

The foregoing example also illustrates a corollary of Hypothesis II, that *stuttering is inversely related to open expressions of aggression consequent to frustration consequent to feeling loss of impact.* This hypothesis is in line with the stutterer's experiencing of his stuttering as an ego-alien act which he performs against his will and over which he has no volitional control. It is as if by having an automatic device, which he cannot operate purposefully, for blocking spoken aggression, he is not only relieved of responsibility for controlling aggressive expressions of frustration about feeling devalued, he is also relieved of the necessity of being aware of these feelings. Stuttering and open expressions of anger apparently do not coexist. The stutterers observed in this report often became more severely blocked as they appeared to become angry, while disclaiming such feelings. Without exception, however, stuttering was not observed when they appeared to lose their tempers completely.

COROLLARY HYPOTHESIS II-2

Another corollary of Hypothesis II is: *moments of stuttering are inversely related to the level of awareness at which the loss of impact is experienced.* We do not have to be aware of what is happening to us in order to experience the fact of our existence from the highest level of cognitive awareness to the lowest level of vegetative functioning. Although we can know in a highly conscious sense much about what we are and what we do, we nevertheless remain unaware of much of our behavior. Consider, for instance, such activities as facial mannerisms, velar movement during speech and peristaltic action in the small intestine. Some of these behaviors can be focused on consciously, others cannot; but we normally are unaware of them all. So it is with the stutterer's feeling of loss of impact. If he does not recognize this feeling, the probability of his responding to it with stuttering is greater than if he is highly cognizant of it. None of the stutterers reported on here recognized a sense of personal devaluation before or during a block. When they were aware of the feeling associated with blocking, it was always in retrospect.

An eighteen-year-old college girl who stuttered with moderate severity illustrates this hypothesis. During the first fifteen sessions her blocks were severe and her body was tense. Her movements and posture appeared stiff and rigid, as if she were controlling everything she did. Although she recognized the tension and found it unpleasant, she was unable to relax and unable to ascertain why she felt on guard. Prior to her eleventh session she had cried throughout a church service for no reason she could determine, but on later reflection she recalled feeling hopeless and resigned. As she discussed the incident she thought the significance of it was that she had decided, in a way of which she was unaware at the time, to continue therapy even though she feared becoming involved in her feelings for her clinician. Halfway through the sixteenth session, after having discussed how closed-off she felt and how much the therapist's silence disturbed her, she became silent. This was a new development. She appeared to relax as she leaned back in her chair for the first time and tears welled in her eyes. She spoke briefly, and fluently, to say that she had better leave. She ran from the room. Throughout the next session she was embarrassed, tense, stuttering again, and unable to remember most of the preceding session. During the following one, however, she was again relaxed and fluent. She said that during the earlier silence "I felt that I could trust you to see me as I really am.

A 5924

That's the way I feel now, too, but I'm empty. There's nothing for you to see or admire. That's why I can't stand being open with myself or you or anyone, and that's why I stutter to hide it."

Hypothesis III

The third major hypothesis is that *the stutterer develops at a low level of awareness a fantasied idealized identity which serves in lieu of a realistic identity as a behavioral determinant.* Because the stutterer dreads facing the reality of himself for fear of finding that he is nothing, he preserves his symbolic self with an all-powerful fantasied identity composed of what he dreams he could be. Since the fantasy is not bound by reality he can ascribe to it unlimited potential. Although he distrusts it as a basis for assessing his actual impact value, he nevertheless seeks confirmation of it in supporting feedback from his listeners which, when received, he also distrusts. In other words, he does not trust his idealized potential sufficiently to risk testing it openly for fear of confirming its alternative, a totally devalued identity which is as unrealistic a fantasy as is the idealized one. Regardless of the level of awareness at which he experiences these fantasies he knows that they are not grounded in his performance of tangible deeds. Accordingly, he is unable to accept praise, much as he craves it, as a valid basis for building a realistic identity because he feels that if the truth were known he would be seen as a hollow man. Conversely, he discounts negative opinions as invalid because no one can really know his potential which he feels he has not been able to demonstrate.

COROLLARY HYPOTHESIS III-1

The relationship of these fantasies to stuttering can be formulated as follows: *stuttering occurs when the stutterer anticipates a discrepancy between his idealized and devalued fantasied identities.* The important point to note in this hypothesis is that a realistic identity is not involved in the anticipated discrepancy. This is to say that stuttering is not elicited by a variance between what the stutterer would realistically like to be and what he realistically is. He relates his feeling of loss of impact to the unrealistic anticipation of emptiness which is his only alternative to confirmation of his all-powerful idealized identity. He seems to view speech, as was hypothesized earlier, as the modality with which he can, magically, effect the impact that would fulfill his fantasied potential. Since his speech is blocked through no choice of his own, he is freed of the responsibility of demonstrating what he could be.

A young minister's description of how he felt about speaking and stuttering is relevant to the point. He said, "I feel that I must speak into myself instead of out to others. I go through the motions of talking to people but I don't say anything that's vital. It's as if I talked long enough and said something, I'd drain myself empty. The trouble is I feel compelled by the outside to say something but I can only preserve my feeling of strength by keeping everything inside. I'm afraid to reveal my inner self because people won't think I'm human. When I look at my thoughts inside, they're white and important, but when I speak them they change color to black and they seem so degraded and foolish. It's like I'm constantly painting masterpieces. Of course I know they aren't real masterpieces but they feel like it inside and the only way I can protect them is to spoil them so people won't know for sure that they weren't masterpieces. You know, I just realized that that's what I do to my speech and my ideas when I stutter."

The use of stuttering as a protective device it not without its consequences, however. Roe[2] has pointed out that after a block the stutterer feels shame for having let himself down again by hiding behind the stuttering rather than risking openly a test of what he is in reality. The shame in this analysis is not so much in relation to the social stigma associated with stuttering as it is a consequence of the feeling of weakness and failure symbolized by the block.

COROLLARY HYPOTHESIS III-2

Another corollary hypothesis closely related to the preceding one is, *stuttering varies directly with the stutterer's concern for the listener's recognition of his idealized potential.* This formulation is designed to account for some puzzling manifestations of increased stuttering. Normally, of course, we think of stuttering increasing when the stutterer speaks with persons of authority, but a young bank executive found himself blocking severely with

---

[2]Personal communication with Allison Roe.

his secretaries and clerks while being fluent with his president. He finally detected some feelings that seemed to account for this paradox. His secretaries and clerks, whom he considered to be immensely inferior to himself, were causing him acute frustration by not according him the respect and deference to which he felt entitled from them. By contrast, he felt quite confortable with his president, a distinguished, elderly gentleman, who seemed so far above him that he did not even expect to be noticed, so any recognition by the president was more than he anticipated.

COROLLARY HYPOTHESIS III-3

A condition that is also related to Hypothesis III can be formulated as follows: *stuttering is reduced or absent when the stutterer feels that his listener recognizes his idealized potential.* Communication of this recognition to the stutterer is not easy. Evidence of acceptance that might normally be sufficient in a relationship is apt to be inadequate for the stutterer. In fact, it may be seen as evidence of disinterest or rejection.

> A twenty-eight-year-old writer described the problem well by saying, "I seem to waste affection on people. They're all like stone walls that it has no affect on. I want to like people and I'm very patient with them and try very hard, but they just won't like me. I just can't seem to get their affection and approval, and I have to have it or I can't bear living in reality. But anger really ties me up because it isolates me even farther from people, and because I'm reacting to them so much I can't escape into my inner world. Since I seem to be the only one who feels affection, I see little value in going from my warm private innerself in which I can feel perfect into the cold barren outside world. The only way I can make that shift easily is when I'm in communion with someone who makes me feel that I'm everything in reality that I secretly am inside. Then I don't need any front and everything's O.K. Maybe that's why I'm such a perfectionist. I'm trying to be as perfect in real life as I am in my daydreams in the hope that people will be impressed and give me the approval I need."

COROLLARY HYPOTHESIS III-4

The alternative to the preceding hypothesis is: *stuttering is reduced or absent when the stutterer views himself entirely within the devalued identity.* The suspicion is strong that blocking occurs only when the stutterer is struggling to live with his idealized and devalued images simultaneously. If he is entirely within himself, he can preserve whatever picture of perfection he may choose in fantasy, hence, no struggle and no stuttering. Conversely, if he views himself entirely within the devalued image, he abandons hope and is, surprisingly, equally free from struggle and stuttering despite his misery and depression. An accountant who has never blocked with his subordinates but had always had difficulty with his supervisors suddenly reversed this pattern. A month earlier a new supervisor had taken over and had insisted on everything being done according to his specifications. As the accountant reported, "I finally reached the point last week where I gave up. I know this guy isn't going to listen to me regardless of how good my reasons are for doing it my way. When I'm talking to him I feel just like a useless blob on the floor, but for some reason I don't stutter anymore with him. The people working under me never used to bother me when we were doing things my way, but now when I have to tell them to do things his way I get all tied up."

The world the stutterer has built for himself seems to be a consequence of his fear of asserting himself with overt deeds. To the extent that he is dependent on the approval of others, he must conform to what he feels would make an impact on them—perfect performance in keeping with his idealized potential. Accordingly, he is paralyzed in his efforts to perform; he cannot run the risk of failure so he must live with his dreams of what he could be rather than with the satisfaction of what he is. Those stutterers reported on here who have been the most successful in extricating themselves from this trap, and from their stuttering, are the ones who have run the risk of exposure by asserting themselves openly with tangible acts of which they are proud. As they have begun to establish their identities in reality, they have discovered that this entails a dynamic process of becoming what they want to be that is distinctly different from the static notion they held, a notion that all of their problems would be over if they could somehow burst forth with their fantasied potential fully realized. Although their realistic goals have often contained elements of the fantasies, they have been, for the most part, of less heroic, more modest dimensions. Ironically, as these stutterers have found satisfaction in the fallible business of humble human accomplishment, not only has their stuttering and the magical power of speech diminished but their idealized and devalued images have withered away from disuse.

References

Bloodstein, O.: The development of stuttering: II Developmental phases. *J. Speech Hearing Dis., 25*:366-376, 1960.

Goodstein, Leonard D.: Functional speech disorders and personality: a survey of the research. *J. Speech Hearing Res., 1*:359-376, 1958.

Hayakawa, S. I.: Conditions of success in communication. *Bull. Menninger Clin., 26*:225-236, 1962.

Sheehan, Joseph G.: Projection studies of stuttering. *J. Speech Hearing Dis., 23*:18-25, 1958.

St. Onge, K. R.: The stuttering syndrome. *J. Speech Hearing Dis., 6*:195-197, 1963.

Teilhard de Chardin, P.: *The Phenomenon of Man.* New York, Harper & Row, 1961.

Trotter, W. D. and Bergmann, M. F.: Stutterers' and non-stutterers' reactions to speech situations. *J. Speech Hearing Dis., 22*:40-45, 1957.

Wingate, M. E.: Evaluation and stuttering: III. Identification of stuttering and the use of a label. *J. Speech Hearing Dis., 27*:368-377, 1962.

3

Stuttering as an Outgrowth of Normal Disfluency

Oliver Bloodstein, Ph.D.
Janice P. Alper, M.A.
Paulette Kendler Zisk, M.A.

I t is well known that most normal young children exhibit a relatively large amount of interruption in their speech of many types. When we consider the question of how such "normal disfluency" is related to stuttering we have the choice of several hypotheses. First, there may be no relationship at all. A good many theories of stuttering have been proposed which substantially ignore the phenomenon of normal disfluency. Second, stuttering may represent the attempt to avoid normal disfluency. This is the "diagnosogenic" theory as originally advanced by Johnson (1942). A third concept, which forms the subject of this contribution, is that stuttering as a clinical disorder is simply an exaggeration or extension of certain kinds of disfluency to be heard in the speech of normal children. This viewpoint has begun to find outspoken expression only in recent years (Bloodstein, 1961; Shames and Sherrick, 1963), although it is implicit in certain earlier writings (e.g. Métraux, 1950) in which the normally disfluent speech of children was referred to as "stuttering" without excessive concern for the need to draw a distinct line between the "normal" and the "abnormal." The question at issue

31

is a pivotal one, since the choice of several major points of view currently held about the onset of stuttering hinges on the manner in which stuttering and normal disfluency are related. The purpose of this chapter is to discuss stuttering as a phenomenon essentially continuous with normal disfluency and to present some research findings which appear to support this hypothesis.

Some Basic Considerations

Stuttering as an Anticipatory Struggle Reaction

There is a concept about the nature of stuttering behavior, which may be termed the *anticipatory struggle* concept, that appears to dominate the thinking of contemporary workers who specialize in the scientific study of stuttering. It has been formulated by many writers in various ways (e.g., Johnson and Knott, 1936; Van Riper, 1937; Wischner, 1952; Sheehan, 1953; Bloodstein, 1958; Mysak, 1960, etc.). The unifying assumption of these formulations is that the immediate reason the stutterer blocks on a given word is his expectation that he will have difficulty with it. Having anticipated some kind of failure in his attempt on the word, he tends to attack it with so much force and such elaborate precautions that he could not possibly say it normally. Moreover, the more frequently he fails to say the word properly the more confirmed he becomes in his conviction that he is unable to do so, and so the more he fails.

Numerous items of evidence may be arrayed in support of this concept (Bloodstein, 1959, pp. 45-48). One of the most important of these is the phenomenon of anticipation. As is well known, developed stuttering tends to be accompanied by a process of more or less anxious expectancy of stuttering which is sufficiently vivid so that most adult stutterers are able to predict the occurrence of most of their blocks. It is difficult indeed to account for this ability unless one assumes that it is the anticipation which in some manner causes the stuttering block.

The question of how anticipatory struggle reactions arise is fundamentally the question of how children learn to anticipate difficulties in their speech. The two answers to this question which have had wide currency in recent decades are embodied in Bluemel's concept of primary and secondary stuttering (1932), and in Johnson's "diagnosogenic" theory, later refined as his "interaction" theory of stuttering (1959, Chap. 10). The relative merits of the views that anticipatory struggle reactions develop through fear of "primary" stuttering on the one hand or "normal nonfluency" on the other have been debated at length. The crucial fact to be stressed from the point of view of this discussion is that these two theories have in common a rather unique assumption which has strongly influenced much of our thinking about stuttering. This is the assumption that anticipatory struggle reactions. are to be distinguished sharply and categorically from "simpler" forms of speech interruption, and that the one arises exclusively as a reaction of avoidance of the other. In a basic sense it is this mold of thought and its implications which form much of the subject matter of this chapter.

The Consistency Effect as a Feature of Anticipatory Struggle Behavior

To an appreciable extent the issue with which we will be concerned hinges on the meaning of the so-called "consistency" effect in stuttering. It is known that in successive oral readings of the same passage a given stutterer tends to block at the same points in the speech sequence at which he has had difficulty before (Johnson and Knott, 1937). That is, stutterings are apparently not distributed in a haphazard fashion, but occur as a response to stimuli. The consistency effect would appear to signify that for every person who stutters there are specific features of the speech sequence which come to serve as "cues" eliciting the expectation of stuttering. These cues may take the form of words, sounds, positions in the sentence, grammatical parts of speech, or other aspects of the context (Brown, 1945). They seem to acquire the, power to evoke expectancy because the stutterer is likely to regard them as difficult or conspicuous, or because they come to remind him of past failures in speech.

A very significant inference which may be drawn from this is that whenever the consistency effect is observed in stuttering it may be taken as indirect evidence of the process of anticipation which is in operation. The consistency effect may consequently be said to be a basic identifying feature of anticipatory struggle reactions.

A Study of the Consistency Effect in Normal Disfluency

In a recent study (Bloodstein, 1960) the consistency effect was found to be a common characteristic of the repetitions and prolongations of a group of young stuttering children. If the inferences we have drawn about the consistency effect are correct this would appear to be an interesting and from certain points of view unexpected finding, because it would seem to imply that what has often been referred to as "primary" stuttering is actually anticipatory struggle behavior, not inherently different from more advanced forms of stuttering except in degree.

Findings such as these occasion considerable wonder about the extent to which the consistency effect is to be found in so-called "normal" disfluencies as well. We quote from the publication in which this study was reported:

> Considerable evidence has been presented to support the view that even the simplest reiterations of the youngest [stuttering] child may be true anticipatory struggle reactions from the point of view of the attitudes and assumptions which underlie them. If this is so, then the problem which at first glance seems to arise is how to distinguish between the repetitions of stuttering and those which are normal for young children to have, since it can hardly be denied that, with all of their similarity to advanced stuttering, some of the symptoms of Phase One* also bear striking resemblances to normal nonfluency. On what basis were Phase One repetitions identified as stutterings? The answer is, chiefly on the evidence of the consistency effect which marked them as anticipatory struggle reactions. Would it, then, be correct to say that stutterings exhibit the consistency effect while normal nonfluencies do not? It would certainly be convenient to be able on the basis of such a simple diagnostic test to say that this child is 'normal' while that child is not. There is, however, one important condition which must first be met. It is necessary to show that the consistency effect is not found in the hesitancies of children who are regarded as normal speakers (Bloodstein, 1961).

---

*In the publication from which this is quoted the course of development of stuttering was discussed as a process involving essentially four phases, Phase One representing the incipient form of the disorder as chiefly found in preschool children.

It was this thinking which prompted the investigation with which we are concerned here.*

Procedure

The subjects were ten children enrolled in a private school in Brooklyn.** They consisted of six boys and four girls ranging in age from four years and five months to six years and six months, with a median age of five years and four months. Six were white and four Negro, this division reflecting in a general way the racial composition of the school's enrollment. The ten subjects were selected from a larger group of twenty-seven pupils by means of a screening test designed to eliminate children who were unable to follow adequately the procedures required by the study or who were too fluent to provide sufficient data. For this purpose each child was instructed to repeat a list of sixteen sentences from dictation twice in succession. Of the children who completed this task eleven exhibited the minimum of eight disfluencies arbitrarily chosen to qualify a child as a subject for the study. One of these subsequently was dropped from the investigation because of poor attendance.

It is to be noted that the subjects were among the more rather than less disfluent of a group of children by virtue of the method by which they were selected. It is clear, however, that they were not in any reasonable sense an extraordinary or highly selected group with respect to the bases on which they were screened. All were regarded as normal speakers by both their parents and their teachers. All had been noted by their teachers to be "average" in intelligence with the exception of one child who was considered "above average."

The experimental testing material consisted of five parts. Four of these were lists of ten sentences each. The fifth part consisted of nursery rhyme material containing twenty-four short lines of verse. The total number of words contained in the material was four hundred and seventy-eight. In the case of one subject who

*This study was done as a Brooklyn College Masters thesis research project by Janice P. Alper and Paulette Kendler Zisk under the direction of Oliver Bloodstein. For a more detailed report of the study see Pearlstein (1962) and Zisk (1962).

**The cooperation and assistance of Mrs. Gertrude Goldstein, director of the Woodward School, are gratefully acknowledged.

refused to recite nursery rhymes (R. E.) the total number of words actually dictated was three hundred and fifty-four.

Each subject was tested individually in a small quiet room. The procedure followed was to dictate each part of the testing material to the child twice in succession, pausing after every sentence (or line of verse) for the child to repeat it aloud. All of the subject's responses were recorded on a portable tape recorder. In addition, the experimenter made an on-the-spot record of each disfluency observed on a mimeographed copy of the material. Each subject was tested on successive occasions over a period of several weeks. His two repetitions of a given part of the material, however, were in each case completed in immediate succession on a single occasion.

A verbatim transcript of each subject's responses was made, and his disfluencies were identified. Six types of disfluency were studied in this investigation: 1) syllable (or sound) repetition; 2) word repetition; 3) phrase repetition; 4) prolongation of sound; 5) interjection, and 6) revision.

By suitable methods it was determined that both experimenters were reliable observers of disfluency.

Results and Interpretations

As in most previous research and clinical work on the consistency effect, the measure employed in this study was the percentage of consistency (Johnson, Darley and Spriestersbach, 1963, p. 274). That is, the words pronounced disfluently by the subject in all of his second repetitions from dictation were identified, and it was then determined what percentage of these words had also been pronounced disfluently on the first dictation. For this purpose all of the test material was considered *in toto* for each subject as though it were a single four hundred and seventy-eight word passage read twice in succession.

The principal findings are summarized in Table I. In the line headed *P.C. Total Disfluency* it will be seen that the percentages of consistency of the ten subjects for disfluency as a whole ranged from 11.1 to 40.0. In an absolute sense these percentages are not large. For example, in a study mentioned above Bloodstein (1960) found percentages of consistency ranging from 50 to 100 for a

TABLE I

MEASURES OF CONSISTENCY OF DISFLUENCY OF TEN SUBJECTS
IN TWO SUCCESSIVE REPETITIONS OF DICTATED MATERIAL

	Subjects									
	B.E.	R.W.	M.A.	C.R.	L.B.	G.H.	K.F.	E.R.	L.T.	R.E.
P.C.* Total disfluency	35.0	13.3	12.5	33.3	23.8	20.0	11.1	18.5	40.0	37.9
Initial percentage of disfluency	4.8	3.4	1.7	4.8	3.4	2.5	4.6	3.1	3.8	10.7
z	2.82	1.13	0.92	2.34	2.20	1.38	0.88	2.06	3.29	3.02
P	.01	NS	NS	.05	.05	NS	NS	.05	.01	.01
P.C. Syllable repetitions	33.3	16.7	33.3	25.0	28.6	0.0	0.0	28.6	42.9	42.9
P.C. Word repetitions	100.0	25.0	—**	100.0	20.0	50.0	0.0	33.3	25.0	36.4
P.C. Phrase repetitions	—	0.0	0.0	100.0	0.0	0.0	50.0	0.0	100.0	0.0
P.C. Prolongations	0.0	—	—	0.0	50.0	—	0.0	0.0	0.0	—
P.C. Revisions	30.8	0.0	0.0	0.0	25.0	50.0	0.0	22.2	75.0	0.0
P.C. Interjections	100.0	—	0.0	50.0	—	0.0	—	0.0	0.0	66.6

*Percentage of consistency.

**No percentage of consistency could be computed in those cases in which a given type of disfluency did not occur during the second repetition of the material.

group of young stutterers tested by methods similar to the ones used here. It must be recalled, however, that a characteristic of the percentage measure of consistency as it is ordinarily computed is that its size is dependent on the initial frequency of stuttering. (See Tate and Cullinan, 1962.) It is not difficult to see why this is so. If all the words of a passage are stuttered in the initial reading, then 100 per cent of the stuttering in any subsequent reading most inevitably occur on words which were stuttered initially. On the other hand, if no words are stuttered at all in the first reading the percentage of consistency cannot be anything but zero. Chiefly for this reason,* any conclusion about degree of consistency of disfluency must be drawn with careful regard for the initial number of disfluencies. In this case these initial frequencies were unusually small (see the second line of Table I), as we would expect when dealing with normal disfluencies. We must conclude that there is little to be learned from a direct comparison of the obtained percentages of consistency with those

---

*And also because Tate and Cullinan (1962) have shown that consistency and initial frequency of stuttering seem to be related even when allowances are made for this peculiarity of the percentage measure.

which have usually been computed for stutterers. The only question which we may meaningfully ask about these percentages is to what extent they exceed values which would be expected by chance alone.

This question is readily answered. Johnson and Knott (1937) have pointed out that the percentage of consistency to be expected on the basis of chance alone is equal to the *initial percentage of stuttering.* "Suppose, for example, one stutters 10 per cent of all the words in the first reading of a passage. Now, in the second reading of the passage he is no more likely *by chance* to stutter on one word than on any other word. Therefore, *by chance* 10 per cent of the words he stutters in the second reading will be among the 10 per cent that he stuttered in the first reading . . ." (Johnson, Darley and Spriesterbach, 1963, p. 275). Consequently, each percentage of consistency in the first line of Table I is to be compared with the percentage in the line just below. It will be seen that the measure of consistency considerably exceeds the initial percentage of disfluency in every case. The two succeeding lines of Table I show that this difference was statistically significant for six of the ten subjects.

The six significant differences, and the near-significance of two others, serve to raise the question of whether the failure of some of the measures to achieve significance was not due chiefly to the exceedingly small amount of disfluency which was observed on the second dictation in those instances. All that we can say for certain is that further confirmation by means of research with larger amounts of test material will be necessary before we can assume that essentially all children exhibit the consistency effect in their normal disfluencies beyond chance expectation. Even to demonstrate the consistency effect in six out of ten subjects, however, is to show that the phenomenon appears at the very least to be quite common in the speech of normal young children.

When we go on to consider the consistency effect in relation to specific types of disfluency we are confronted by a choice between two possible ways to define what we are talking about. As an illustration, each value shown for *word repetition* in Table I represents the percentage of repeated words on the second dictation which the subject had pronounced disfluently *in any way* on the first dictation. The values would have been distinctly smaller if we had insisted that the disfluencies be identical in type on both dictations to qualify as instances of consistency. Neither of these definitions is more valid than the other, but the second is considerably more exacting than the first, and would compel us to overlook many instances of coincident disfluency which presumably are not mere chance occurrences. Perhaps the chief justification for defining consistency as we have done in Table I is that in none of the past research on the consistency effect in stuttering to which the present study is essentially parallel has there been the requirement that the symptoms in any sense duplicate themselves.

As Table I shows, consistency appeared to some extent in every category of disfluency. But the outstanding finding with respect to these specific categories was the apparent tendency for repetitions, particularly of syllables and words, to be distributed consistently more often than other types of disfluency. The amounts of disfluency, when subdivided in this way, were too small to permit meaningful statistical tests, but the data in Table I seems to reflect a trend which is difficult to ignore. If valid, this finding is interesting in view of the frequency with which word and syllable repetitions have been identified as early symptoms of stuttering.

The Continuity of Stuttering and Normal Disfluency

Normal Disfluency as Anticipatory Struggle Behavior

We have reported a study which appears to afford evidence that the consistency effect, which has heretofore been investigated in the context of stuttering, is also in some measure a feature of normal speech hesitancy in at least certain of its aspects. How is this to be interpreted? One obvious explanation is that the consistency effect is not the major distinguishing feature of anticipatory struggle behavior in speech that we have thought it to be, despite all the apparent evidence to the contrary as summarized earlier, and deserves to be ignored. There is, however, another interpretation which should be considered carefully.

The possibility needs to be pondered that some of what we call "normal childhood nonfluency" consists of true anticipatory struggle reactions in the sense that they are based on the child's evaluation of the word, or phrase, or sentence of the moment as difficult to say, on his expectation that without unusual effort he may fail to pronounce or articulate it acceptably, and in a general way on the subtle aura of formidability which speech is likely to possess for someone who is still a novice in its rituals, strictures and taboos. If so, then the speech behavior which we call stuttering may not differ fundamentally except in degree from certain types of behavior which we refer to as normal disfluency. This basic premise was expressed in an earlier publication (Bloodstein, 1961) as follows:

> . . . it seems an extremely plausible assumption that the reason the symptoms of some children referred to the speech clinic do not contrast sharply with the hesitations of many normal youngsters is that anticipatory struggle behavior is characteristic to some degree of the speech of almost all young children. It would be rather curious if this were not so. One may be fairly sure that the influences which produce stuttering are present to a small extent in almost every child's environment. Consequently, almost every child can be expected to exhibit mildly and fleetingly the tensions and fragmentations which develop into identifiable episodes of stuttering in a few . . .
>
> Ever since such a thing as normal nonfluency was recognized, it appears to have been assumed that it was something to be distinguished categorically from "stuttering." This has given rise to one of the most taxing problems with which speech clinicians have been beset in recent years—the problem of determining what, precisely, is the difference between the two, and of making a judgment in the speech clinic as to whether a given pattern of speech interruptions in a young child is or is not "stuttering." Actually, it appears to be far more natural to assume that there exists only a difference of degree between the normal and abnormal. In all probability, the question of how to differentiate between stuttering and normal nonfluency can never have an absolute answer. The only distinction which one can validly make appears to be a purely relative one between struggle reactions which are mild and occasional and those which are more severe and persistent.

One has only to consider the insoluble problems with which psychotherapists would be faced if they insisted on making a sharp distinction between "neurotic" and "normal" individuals to appreciate how implausible may be the assumptions on which we have been attempting to operate in the area of stuttering. Aside from its *a priori* appeal, however, the assumption that stuttering is continuous with certain forms of normal disfluency is supported by a number of other facts and observations.

The Pervasiveness of Stuttering in Childhood

In the first place, stuttering appears to be prevalent in our society, particularly among children, to a degree which perhaps is seldom suspected. It is well known on the basis of repeated studies that about one per cent of the total population "stutters." This figure in all probability excludes an indeterminate number of mild, occasional, and covert stutterers which may be exceedingly large. What is even more important, however, is that it represents only the incidence of hard core stuttering at a given moment in time. Stuttering frequently appears in children in the form of episodes of weeks, months, or years. So many stutterers appear to "outgrow" their speech difficulty that it is often regarded as primarily a disorder of childhood. Consequently, when we ask a group of individuals to say, not whether they stutter, but whether they have had such a problem *at one time or another,* the incidence is considerably higher than one per cent. Voelker (1942) found that of ninety-six college students 10 per cent replied "yes" to the question, "Did you ever have a stuttering defect of speech?" Villarreal (1945), replicating this study with two hundred and seventy-one subjects, received an affirmative answer to the same question from 14 per cent. Hertzman (1948) found an incidence of about 13 per cent with past histories of stuttering in a questionnaire survey of one thousand eight hundred high school juniors and seniors in Cincinnati.

It is to be further considered that these percentages are confined largely to the type of stuttering episode which is sufficiently protracted or severe to be remembered years afterward. During the early preschool years when most major stuttering problems get their start there appears to be a rather widespread outbreak of mild, transient episodes which are not likely to be recalled by the children themselves later. Data gathered by Glasner and

Rosenthal (1957) on nine hundred and ninety-six children entering the first grade of elementary school in Anne Arundel County, Maryland, show that slightly over 20 per cent were considered by the parents either to be stuttering or to have stuttered at some time in the relatively brief span of time between the onset of speech and first grade registration.

Even these data, moreover, do not take into account the possibility that there may be episodes of stuttering so minor and ephemeral that they are never definitely identified as such by the parents. In this connection it is instructive to study that portion of the findings of Johnson and his associates (1959, pp. 145, 146; Appendix A, pp. 79, 80) which was concerned with the disfluencies of one hundred and fifty normal children. Despite the fact that any children who had ever previously been regarded by their parents as stutterers *had been carefully excluded from the group,* of eighty-four mothers and seventy-five fathers who had noticed nonfluencies in their children's speech approximately one out of six reported in personal interviews that there was some degree of "force" or "effort" or "tension" in the first nonfluencies which they had noticed, and 14 per cent of the fathers and 6 per cent of the mothers reported force or tension at the time of the interview. Furthermore, concerning the child's reaction to his earliest nonfluencies twelve mothers and nine fathers of normal children said that the child seemed to be "aware of the fact that he was speaking in a different manner or doing something wrong"; three mothers and three fathers reported that the child showed "surprise or bewilderment after having had trouble on a word"; seven mothers and three fathers said that the first stoppages seemed to be "unpleasant to the child"; and nine mothers and seven fathers thought that the child "felt irritated" when the first stoppages occurred.

Clearly, to insist that such stoppages are "really" stutterings because of the effort and emotion which accompany them, or to insist that they are "really" normal disfluencies because the parents have not regarded them as anything else is in either case to beg the question. In the theoretical context which we have adopted such a distinction is not crucially significant. We may interpret Johnson's data as well as the evidences we have cited of the widespread incidence of stuttering as showing that from certain points of view stuttering in children is so pervasive a phenomenon as to border on the ordinary and usual, and the more assiduously we press the attempt to establish its exact dimensions the more they seem to merge with the larger outlines of what we generally refer to as "normal" childhood speech hesitancy.

The "Overlapping" of Judgments of Stuttering and Normal Disfluency

This leads to a related kind of observation which has a bearing on our hypothesis. Johnson and his co-workers at the University of Iowa (1959, pp. 132-149) have collected extensive data on the terms which parents of young stutterers use or accept to describe the first speech interruptions which they regard as stuttering in their children, and have compared these with the descriptive terms which parents of nonstutterers use or accept for their children's earliest disfluencies. On a group basis there are distinct differences in these descriptions. Sound or syllable repetitions and prolongations of sounds were reported considerably more often for stutterers, while phrase repetitions, pauses, and interjections of extraneous sounds were reported considerably more often for nonstutterers. Moreover, the earliest stutterings were more often reported to have some degree of "force" or "effort" than the nonstutterers' earliest disfluencies. A notable aspect of the findings, however, was the "overlapping" of the experimental and control groups with respect to these descriptions. There were many children in both groups for whom the descriptive terms were limited to repetitions of syllables, words, or phrases. And, while in some instances the earliest stutterings were said to have been marked by signs of tension and concern or "emotion," the same was true of some of the nonstutterers, as has already been seen.

Furthermore, when tape recorded samples of the speech of the stutterers, made on an average of eighteen months after the reported onset of the problem, were compared with recorded samples of the nonstutterers' speech, analysis again revealed substantial overlapping between the two groups with respect to frequency of disfluencies (Johnson, 1959, pp. 196-220). As a group the stutterers averaged a good deal more sound or syllable repetitions and word repetitions, and somewhat more phrase repetitions and prolonged sounds. But 20 per cent of the male nonstutterers exhibited more overall disfluencies than did 30 per cent of the male stutterers. Even with respect to the types of disfluency which particularly differentiated the two groups it was found that approximately 20 per cent of the male nonstutterers had more sound or syllable repetitions than did 20 per cent of the male stutterers, and 20 per cent of the male nonstutterers repeated words more often than did 20 per cent of the male stutterers. The findings for the female subjects were essentially the same.

In the face of this overlap between the observable features of what has been judged to be "stuttering" and certain observable aspects of what has been judged to be "normal" speech, it would appear to be essentially impossible, as Johnson has pointed out, to formulate a definition of stuttering as a feature of a child's speech which would serve to differentiate it in an operationally meaningful way from normal disfluency. Johnson has interpreted this to mean that stuttering is not to be defined meaningfully as a feature of a person's speech at all, but rather as a "perceptual and evaluative problem" that first arises for a listener as the result of an interaction between the listener and the speaker (1959, pp. 236-264). There is, however, a different interpretation for which it is possible to find support in the data cited from the Iowa onset studies. It may be that the reason the data do not permit us to distinguish what we generally call stuttering operationally from normal disfluencies in any sharp way is simply that they are not wholly or in every respect different things.

An analogy will serve to amplify this interpretation. We tend to define the symptoms of cerebral palsy unhesitatingly as features of a person's behavior, and the question of whether they would be better defined in some other way never seems to come up. Yet, if we were to make detailed observations of the gait, posture, and manual and bodily coordination of a group of so-called "normal" children it is virtually a foregone conclusion that almost any aspect of jerkiness, stiffness, clumsiness, weakness, associated involuntary

activity, or lack of motor control that can be defined or classi-
fied would be exhibited by some "normal" children in greater
measure than by some members of a "cerebral palsied" group,
and it seems highly probable that some of the most poorly coordinated "normal" children would from time to time appear more awkward and clumsy as a whole than some of the more mildly affected
cases of what the neurologist refers to as cerebral palsy. And when
we consider that "normal" clumsiness, like cerebral palsy as a clinical disorder, must always in some way be related to the functioning of the motor centers of the central nervous system, and probably even finds some of its origin in brain injuries associated with
the "normal" birth process, the analogy takes on all the more
relevance. The point is that the overlap which exists between
"normal" and "abnormal" functioning on the level of direct observation of behavior appears to create little difficulty in the definition of cerebral palsy, any more than it does in the definition of
neurotic disorders, infantile articulation, or innumerable other
conditions which we tend to place in more or less distinct contrast with the normal. We adopt such distinctions on a rather
high level of generalization as useful abstractions, and employ
them most effectively with a wholesome awareness that on the
level of direct observation the contrasts are somewhat blurred.

In a similar sense stuttering may be differentiated from normal
disfluency. An abstract concept of stuttering as an abnormal form
of behavior as opposed in a general way to more ordinary kinds
of speech hesitancy is, of course, a useful one, and we will almost
certainly develop indices of disfluency, based on suitable norms
and taking into account the frequency, type, persistence and severity of a child's speech interruptions, the conditions under which
they occur, the age of the child, and so forth, on the basis of which
we will be able to make rough evaluative judgments about the
clinical significance or non-significance of a child's anticipatory
struggle reactions. The point of this discussion is simply that it
is not to be imagined that any line of demarcation drawn in this
way between what is and is not "stuttering" can ever be more than
essentially arbitrary. If we can accept this outlook with regard to
stuttering as we accept it in relation to so many other problems,
there appears to be no special difficulty about defining stuttering

as a feature of a person's speech, dependent on the listener only to the extent that from a broad philosophical point of view all experience is a joint product of the observer and the observed.*

The Sources of Anticipatory Struggle Behavior

We have reviewed several reasons for believing in the concept of a continuum of anticipatory struggle reactions along which severe, chronic stuttering merges by fine degrees with certain forms of normal disfluency. In justifying this concept earlier we suggested that it was only reasonable to assume that the environmental influences which caused major anticipatory struggle reactions in some children were present in at least small degrees in the experience of the majority of children. It is necessary to consider what some of these influences might be.

The basic question which we are discussing is the question of how children learn to behave in varying degrees on the basis of a belief in the difficulty of speech. It was pointed out at the outset of this chapter that two principal views have been held about the answer to this question, one embodied in the concept of primary and secondary stuttering, and the other in Johnson's "diagnosogenic" theory. The first of these says, in effect, that it is chiefly the abnormal amount of disfluency in a child's speech which brings on the parental penalties which foster the conception that acceptable speech requires effort and strain. The second says that it is not the child's unusual disfluencies but the parents' abnormal evaluations of his disfluency which are chiefly to blame. It is clear that in either view anticipatory struggle reactions are seen as attempts to avoid disfluencies, whether "normal" or "abnormal." It is in a sense remarkable that this is so. If we wrestle for a time with the question of which outlook is the more valid another question is likely to obtrude itself. Why is it necessary to assume

---

*This is an appropriate context in which to state the rather obvious fact that to a large extent the viewpoint elaborated in this chapter represents one possible outgrowth of Johnson's theoretical approach to the problem of stuttering, and consequently owes much to it. The "diagnosogenic" theory has served as a sustained focus of therapy and research for over twenty years, and has received wide support, including the ultimate tribute of a lengthy scholarly refutation in a recent volume of a learned journal (Wingate, 1962a, 1962b, 1962c). This chapter is one of many possible examples of the impact which Johnson's thinking has had.

that, except for fluency, no other aspect of speech may serve as a sufficient focus of concern to produce the troublesome expectations of speech failure which underlie anticipatory struggle reactions? It would seem, on the contrary, that there are imperfections of many other kinds in children's speech which might be capable of provoking a considerable amount of parental penalty. Furthermore, there appears to be abundant evidence in clinical observations on young stutterers that such factors often do play a very important part in the onset of the disorder.

A detailed documentation of this viewpoint based on clinical studies of one hundred and eight stuttering children has been presented elsewhere (Bloodstein, 1958). Such case studies divulge an unexpected variety of sources from which a child may acquire a handicapping belief in the difficulty of speech. Broadly speaking, these sources are of three kinds.

In the first place, there are various experiences of failure in speech or language, in addition to excessive hesitancy, which appear capable under certain conditions of instilling in a child a more or less habitual anticipation of speech difficulty. The foremost of these, in relation to the frequency with which they seem to be associated with the onset of stuttering, are infantile errors of articulation. Other common provocations to stuttering are retarded language development, cluttering, pronunciation difficulties, and reading disability. In addition, we have seen cases in which severe dysphonia, cleft palate speech, cerebral palsy speech, or the difficulties encountered in learning a new language appeared to have served as the major provocations.

Such factors are by no means obvious features of every case. Nor would they generally be likely by themselves to produce stuttering. The child must be assisted to regard them as failures or difficulties by a cooperative environment. A second important source of the stutterer's belief in the difficulty of speech, therefore, are the anxieties and demands focused in most cases by the parents with varying degrees of subtlety on the communicative process. These pressures, like the provocations just mentioned, probably have a very large number of possible origins. Frequently, as Johnson has observed, they appear as perfectionistic child training policies reflecting in slightly exaggerated form the anxious strivings which are commonplace in a competitive society. Sometimes an essentially ordinary naiveté on the part of parents concerning what may be expected of a child seems to play a part. In other instances the pressures come chiefly from competition with siblings who have superior speech or language skills, or from the need to emulate a parent whose speech is unusually rapid, fluent, or cultured, or for various reasons has become a highly valued and exacting model. In some cases the fact that a child has spoken unusually early or well serves in a subtle way to create an atmosphere of heightened expectations with regard to his speech. Sometimes, as Johnson has pointed out, the problem appears to be primarily the anxiety of a stuttering family or parent worried about the possibility that the child might stutter. In still other cases the pressures may not come from the home at all, but from a rigid or chronically impatient teacher.

In addition to these relatively ordinary pressures which are to be found in the general run of cases, there are also markedly neurotic family patterns which tend to foster speech anxieties along with the other personality problems they frequently create. For example, a mother may be abnormally dominating or protective. Or a father may make excessive demands which are based on an immature need to see himself glorified in the achievements of his child. Or a parent's basically obsessive-compulsive personality structure may reflect itself in unrealistically high standards of behavior or anxiety-ridden child training practices.

A third source of the attitudes and beliefs which underlie anticipatory struggle behavior is to be found in many cases in the personality of the child himself, in the form of insecurity, excessive need for approval, dependence, fearfulness, or a low threshold of tolerance for frustration. Such traits are not to be found in all stutterers by any means, but when they are present they serve to make a child especially vulnerable to environmental pressures, and especially quick to accept a concept of himself as a failure — at speech or anything else. One personality pattern which turns up often enough to be noteworthy combines high aspirations, conscientiousness, tense perfectionism, sensitiveness, and an essentially adult concern for the feelings of others.

In summary, case studies of young children who are brought to a speech clinic as stutterers disclose a multitude of influences of various kinds, appearing in different combinations in different cases, which seem to make for the child's indoctrination in the belief that speech is a difficult undertaking which requires effort and elaborate care. The point to be noted about these influences, however, is that most of them are essentially ordinary. The great majority of normal children probably encounter some of them, or influences like them, in varying degrees, as features of their daily experience. This accords with the assumption that anticipatory struggle behavior does not occur on an all-or-none basis, that almost all children are influenced from time to time by expectations of speech failure, and that reactions which might justifiably be called stutterings occur transiently in virtually every child's speech.

Stuttering as Tension and Fragmentation in Speech

It will be surprising indeed if many experienced clinical workers react to the foregoing discussion of some of the possible causes of stuttering with the feeling that they are learning something utterly new. On the level of day-to-day clinical experience, for example, it has probably been observed very widely that children with articulatory difficulties or language problems often have episodes of stuttering when they receive too much speech correction at home, or even in the speech clinic, and that stuttering sometimes emerges from anxiety-laden oral recitation situations in the classroom. It is exceedingly interesting, however, that on a theoretical level it has not been easy to explain how such circumstances might lead directly to the development of anticipatory struggle reactions. We have been trapped by a long-standing assumption that an anticipatory struggle reaction was and could only be an attempt to avoid a repetition or other "simple" nonfluency. There are, however, other ways to elaborate the concept of anticipatory struggle which do not imply that it is an "avoidance" of repetitions or anything else.

One of the more satisfactory ways to do so, from certain points of view, is to describe stuttering as a reaction of tension and fragmentation (Bloodstein, 1961). Everyday experience affords continual evidence that whenever we are faced with the necessity to perform an act which we believe is difficult in circumstances in which a great deal hinges on success, two unusual kinds of behavior are likely to be observed as we initiate the act. One is increased muscular effort. The other is a tendency to fragment the act, i.e., to perform a part of it, and often to do so repeatedly before completing it, in an apparent feeling of helplessness to perform the whole act at once. If stuttering reactions are examined carefully it will be noted that almost all of them involve utterance which is to some degree both tense and fragmented. In a general way, we may say that repetitions most conspicuously exemplify the fragmentation of speech, while tension is usually a more obvious feature of such symptoms of stuttering as prolongation.

One of the outstanding advantages of a concept of this kind is that it liberates us from the restrictive notion that anticipatory struggle behavior is an effort to avoid repetitions. It leaves us free to recognize the contribution which may be made to the onset of such behavior by any source whatever from which a child tends to acquire a conviction that speech presents imposing difficulties. It frees us from the assumption that stuttering as anticipatory struggle behavior may arise only as a reaction to either "primary" stutterings or normal disfluencies. For this reason, and because it permits us to view even the simplest repetitive speech behavior as anticipatory struggle, it tends to break down the barrier which has existed in our thinking between "stuttering" and "normal" forms of speech interruption.

Summary and Conclusions

We have presented a number of different kinds of evidence in support of the viewpoint that stuttering is essentially similar to certain forms of normal disfluency, differing from them in degree more than in kind. First, a study of the consistency effect in the disfluencies of normal children strongly suggests that anticipatory struggle reactions are not confined to the speech of children who stutter in the clinical sense of the term. The data are not extensive enough to warrant conclusive statements about degree of consistency, percentage of children, or kinds of disfluency involved, and more research is needed to answer such questions. But the findings leave little doubt that children are not to be divided categorically into stutterers who exhibit the consistency effect and normal speakers who do not. Second, there is evidence that mild, brief episodes of speech hesitation which is identified as stuttering are so widespread in early childhood as to border imperceptibly on the kind of speech behavior which is ordinarily regarded as normal nonfluency. Third, there appears to be a decided overlap between the kinds of speech hesitancy which are described by parents of stutterers as the earliest symptoms of "stuttering" and the descriptions of early speech hesitations which are given by parents of children who speak "normally." Finally there would seem to be a basic implausibility about any conception of human behavior which separates people in an unqualified way into "normal" and "abnormal."

This viewpoint lends itself to elaboration as a relatively comprehensive theory of the etiology of stuttering. To begin with, speech is by far the most crucial of all interpersonal extensions of ourselves, the most vulnerable to critical scrutiny, and the most liable to become an object of self-conscious fears and inhibitions. Virtually all of us, furthermore, are subject to communicative pressures from a great variety of sources in our social environment. Young children tend to have a somewhat precarious hold on the speech and language habits of their society, and to experience the threat of speech failure comparatively often. They are also particularly accessible to social pressures as mediated by parental attitudes. With these things in mind, we may hypothesize that most if not substantially all children learn to believe on various levels of consciousness, under varying conditions, for varying periods of time, and with widely varying degrees of conviction and concern, in the difficulty of speech; that the majority of children consequently exhibit mild, intermittent tensions and fragmentations in their speech; and that in a relatively small number of cases the pressures, provocations, and other influences at work are so numerous, intense, and long-lasting, and the resulting tensions and fragmentations so persistent and severe, that, with due regard for the arbitrary nature of the judgment involved and for the disagreement about it which would necessarily exist among listeners, the child may be said to be "stuttering."

This is not to say that any and all of the disfluencies which are exhibited by young children are related to what is ordinarily regarded as stuttering. There are many different forms of interruption in children's speech, and it is unlikely that all of them are antici- patory struggle reactions in the sense in which this term has been used here. Our thesis is simply that among the disfluencies to be heard in the speech of nearly all young children there are early prototypes of stuttering behavior which will develop into chronic and troublesome problems in a few cases. On the basis of present knowledge it would appear that among the most notable of the primitive stutterings of normal children are syllable and word repetitions, and prolongations of sound.

In summary we may say that stuttering is an outgrowth of normal disfluency. In the course of its development it often under- goes a considerable process of change as tensions and fragmenta- tions become extreme and devices for circumventing them make their appearance, so that in the end we may fail to recognize in the stuttering behavior its commonplace beginnings. Stuttering ap- pears to be essentially an intensification, an exaggeration, and ul- timately, in its developed forms, a monstrification of certain kinds of normal disfluency. The basic practical implication of this kind of orientation to the problem is that whatever knowledge we gain about normal disfluency in young children is likely to increase our knowledge about the origins, prevention, and early treatment of stuttering, and that the quest for a more adequate understanding of stuttering therefore needs to be pursued in the direction of a better understanding of such disfluency.

References

Bloodstein, O.: The development of stuttering: I. Changes in nine basic features. *J. Speech Hearing Dis., 25*:219-237, 1960.

Bloodstein, O.: The development of stuttering: II. Developmental phases. *J. Speech Hearing Dis., 25*:366-376, 1960a.

Bloodstein, O.: The development of stuttering: III. Theoretical and clinical implications. *J. Speech Hearing Dis., 26*:67-82, 1961.

Bloodstein, O.: *A Handbook on Stuttering for Professional Workers.* Chicago, National Society for Crippled Children and Adults, 1959.

Bloodstein, O.: Stuttering as an anticipatory struggle reaction. In Eisenson, J., ed.: *Stuttering: A Symposium.* New York, Harper & Bros., 1958.

Brown, S. F.: The loci of stutterings in the speech sequence. *J. Speech Dis., 10*:181-192, 1945.

Glasner, P. J. and Rosenthal, D.: Parental diagnosis of stuttering in young children. *J. Speech Hearing Dis., 22*:288-295, 1957.

Hertzman, J.: High school mental hygiene survey. *Amer. J. Orthopsychiat., 18*:238-256, 1948.

Johnson, W.: *The Onset of Stuttering.* Minneapolis, Univ. Minnesota Press, 1959.

Johnson, W., *et al*: A study of the onset and development of stuttering. *J. Speech Dis., 7*:251-257, 1942.

Johnson, W., Darley, F. L. and Spriestersbach, D. C.: *Diagnostic Methods in Speech Pathology.* New York, Harper & Row, 1963.

Johnson, W. and Knott, J. R.: The moment of stuttering. *J. Genet. Psychol., 48*:475-479, 1936.

Johnson, W. and Knott, J. R.: Studies in the psychology of stuttering: I. The distribution of moments of stuttering in successive readings of the same material. *J. Speech Dis., 2*:17-19, 1937.

Métraux, R. W.: Speech profiles of the pre-school child 18 to 54 months. *J. Speech Hearing Dis., 15:* 37-53, 1950.

Mysak, E. D.: Servo theory and stuttering. *J. Speech Hearing Dis., 25*:188-195, 1960.

Pearlstein, J. S.: The consistency effect in the speech revisions, prolongations and interjections of young children. M.A. thesis, Brooklyn College, 1962.

Shames, G. H. and Sherrick, C. E., Jr.: A discussion of nonfluency and stuttering as operant behavior. *J. Speech Hearing Dis., 28*:3-18, 1963.

Sheehan, J. G.: Theory and treatment of stuttering as an approach-avoidance conflict. *J. Psychol., 36*:27-49, 1953.

Tate, M. W. and Cullinan, W. L.: Measurement of consistency of stuttering. *J. Speech Hearing Res., 5*:272-283, 1962.

Van Riper, C.: The preparatory set in stuttering. *J. Speech Dis., 2*:149-154, 1937.

Villarreal, J. J.: The semantic aspects of stuttering in non-stutterers: additional data. *Quart. J. Speech, 31*:477-479, 1945.

Voelker, C. H.: On the semantic aspects of stuttering in non-stutterers. *Quart. J. Speech, 28*:78-80, 1942.

Wingate, M. E.: Evaluation and stuttering: I. Speech characteristics of young children. *J. Speech Hearing Dis., 27*:106-115, 1962a.

Wingate, M. E.: Evaluation and stuttering: II. Environmental stress and critical appraisal of speech. *J. Speech Hearing Dis., 27*:244-257, 1962b.

Wingate, M. E.: Evaluation and stuttering: III. Identification of stuttering and the use of a label. *J. Speech Hearing Dis., 27*:368-377, 1962c.

Wischner, G. J.: An experimental approach to expectancy and anxiety in stuttering behavior. *J. Speech Hearing Dis., 17*:139-154, 1952.

Zisk, P. K.: The consistency effect in the speech repetitions of young children. M.A. thesis, Brooklyn College, 1962.

4

A Discussion of Nonfluency and Stuttering as Operant Behavior*

George H. Shames, Ph.D.
Carl E. Sherrick, Jr., Ph.D.

Within the broad purview of verbal behavior, the phenomenon of stuttering has often been singled out for special attention. Stuttering has for some time been of interest to experimental psychology as a vehicle for studying the function of anxiety in the acquisition of behavior. It has also been of interest to cultural anthropology, semantics, psychoanalysis, and clinical psychology as behavior which can be explained by and structurally embedded within their respective theoretical languages. In addition to these disciplines, there is an increasing number of theorists, researchers, and clinicians who are seeking to resolve and understand stuttering as a clinical problem.

It is the purpose of this paper to discuss procedures for the further study of stuttering as a clinical problem within the framework of operant conditioning. As a procedure for categorizing behavior, operant analysis resembles the procedures of any theory of stuttering by which events are placed in relation to one another. However, operant analysis requires minimal assumptions and

*Reprinted from the *Journal of Speech and Hearing Disorders*, February 1963, Vol. 28, No. 1.

inferences regarding the events which are observed and the principles underlying these events. It is hoped that an improved behavioral analysis of stuttering will eventually provide a better definition of the events grouped under this term. Well-defined and precise observations of individual stuttering histories and of the events before, during, and after specific episodes of current stuttering should help us to arrive at effective methods for experimentally controlling this behavior and, ultimately, to develop techniques for clinical application.

The System of Operant Analysis

Skinner has developed a system of behavioral analysis *(15,* pp. 59-90) which has been demonstrated by Goldiamond *(7,8)* to apply to the problem of stuttering. Operant behavior may be characterized as that behavior by means of which the organism does something to his external environment.

The criterion for deciding whether or not behavior is operant is mainly that its properties may be modified by the effects that result from its appearance. Fundamentally, the system is supposed to stem from a definite pattern of laboratory practices. The subject is trained to behave under certain specified conditions. When the experimenter manipulates these conditions, observations are made of changes in behavior. The events during these controlled observations are categorized into broad classes of stimuli and responses. Some unique relations have been perceived among these classes of stimuli and classes of responses. One such relation is manifest when a given class of responses appears more frequently when followed by one of a set of stimulus classes. These stimuli which appear to increase the frequency of a class of responses that they follow are called positive reinforcers, provided also that their removal reduces the frequency of the response. The weakening or extinction of a response is brought about by removal of the reinforcer. Another relation perceived among responses, and stimuli which follow them, are those stimuli which tend to interrupt or depress responses. This is sometimes referred to as punishment. These stimuli are often thought to be aversive since the subject may increase in frequency those responses which tend to reduce or remove these stimuli. This relation between responses and the termination of ongoing aversive stimuli has been termed negative reinforcement. Both positive and negative reinforcement imply an increased frequency of responses while extinction and punishment imply a weakening of responses.

It has also been observed that certain stimulus events lead to particular responses. Such events do not appear to reinforce behavior; they seem to evoke it These stimuli come to control responses because they have been discriminated as part of the total stimulus occasion when a response has been reinforced. Skinner has designated these as discriminative stimuli. Thus we have Skinner's basic three-term paradigm of $S^D \longrightarrow R \longrightarrow Rf$ representing the contingency of discriminative stimulus, response, and reinforcement.

In selecting from the literature and from past experience the events of stuttering to be viewed through operant analysis, we shall employ many of the dimensions of observation that have proved useful to speech pathology. For convenience, we shall trace with the terms of operant behavior a rough progression of conditioning, beginning with the events associated with non-fluency, through the onset and development of early stuttering, to the events observed in advanced stuttering. These include conditioning with positive reinforcement, with negative reinforcement, or with punishment. By placing our observations of nonfluency and stuttering within these paradigms, we can hypothesize more specifically that stuttering responses are under the control of specific discriminative stimuli, aversive stimuli, or other reinforcing contingencies. Past clinical observation and experience directs and restricts the selection to a limited number of stimuli and contingencies that will be discussd in this paper. The ultimate relevance of these stimuli to the responses classed as stuttering can be determined only through experimentation and observation. It is felt that as experimental analyses proceed, many other contingencies will emerge that may have more subtle application to both clinical and theoretical aspects of stuttering. These, of course, are beyond the scope of the present paper.

Nonfluency

Studies by Davis *(4, 5, 6)* and Winitz *(18)* have suggested that speech nonfluencies in such diverse forms as repetitions, prolongations, interjections, and pauses have a high operant level in children. Repetition has been the most frequently observed form as the repetition of codified speech is a part of the child's repertoire by the age of two.

The conditions surrounding the original emission and early development of nonfluencies in the speech of infants are still quite obscure and in need of detailed observation. It is possible that the repetitions observed in later speech may be related to the vocal behavior emitted by infants during their early speech development (babbling and chaining of syllables). Winitz (18) offers data which can be interpreted to support such a hypothesis. It is also possible that nonfluency in speech is a characteristic of the human organism because of its physiological limitations. Speech is an adjunctive function of organs having basically biological functions. As such, speech appears within the limitations of these other functions; we must, for example, pause and hesitate if only to inhale.

In addition to the possibility of such biological origins, many observations of the modification of nonfluency suggest several hypotheses regarding the conditioning of nonfluency that should also be submitted to analysis. It has been observed that the verbal behavior of a speaker varies due to relatively simple acts by his listener. Many of these acts are such signs of attention as looking, nodding, smiling, or speaking. We infer that these listener activities are positive reinforcers because we observe that the speaker continues to speak as long as these activitis continue. Moreover, the speaker's behavior may diminish in strength when these listener activities are no longer forthcoming. Such positive reinforcements not only maintain verbal behavior; they are a part of the basis for conditioning verbal behavior.

It is possible to view the repetition response as a class of verbal responses with a history of complex schedules of reinforcement. The initial appearance of repetition may have a basis that is entirely foreign to its development as nonfluency. For example, we frequently repeat to make sure that a listener has heard us correctly. On several occasions of a repetition having this basis, the speaker is reinforced by the listener for repetitions and not for single utterances. On future occasions the likelihood of repetitions may then become greater than that of single utterances.

States of Deprivation and Aversive Stimuli

The studies of Davis *(4, 5, 6)*, in addition to suggesting the relation of age to the strength and forms of nonfluent speech, have also suggested the occasions for their emission in specific situations. She observed that repetitions, which were the commonest form of nonfluency, seemed to be related to getting attention, directing someone else's activities, trying to gain an object, coercion, seeking status, giving and seeking information, criticizing, seeking a privilege, and trying to obtain social acceptance.

It is interesting to note that nearly all of these occasions involve a type of verbal behavior which Skinner calls "manding" *(16)*, p. 35). This type of verbal behavior is often in the interrogative or imperative mood and is controlled by the listener's positive reinforcements on the occasion of an aversive stimulus or a specific state of deprivation in the speaker. Typically the listener does something for the speaker or gives something to the speaker. The listener's behavior can have the effect of increasing the likelihood of a particular form of verbal behavior by the speaker on future occasions of similar aversive stimuli or deprivations. An example would be the young child who says, "Teacher, look!" followed by the teacher giving her attention to the child by "looking." The child in essence has indicated to the teacher the form of reinforcement for his utterance, "Teacher, look!" In the future, if the child wants the teacher's attention, he may emit the same form of verbal behavior.

Davis's observations suggest that a relation between repetition responses and occasions of aversive stimuli or states of deprivation should be studied. Such manding behavior by the child is on a haphazard schedule of reinforcement; the demands of the child are not always reinforced by parents and peers. If repetitions are frequently connected with the variable reinforcement of these demands, the repetition will then appear in greater strength, since they are being reinforced on the same schedule as the child's manding. An example might be the parent who delays reinforcement of a child's first utterance because of the inconvenience of providing the reinforcement. The child may then repeat the utterance several times, until the repetition becomes undesirable to the parent. The parent finally provides positive reinforcement for the child's demands, perhaps unaware that he is not only doing something for his child but is also *teaching him to repeat*. If we extend this example to consider some future behavior of the parent, we may eventually see some etiological relations among: a) the inconvenience of reinforcing his child's manding; b) a connection between the child's repetition and this inconvenience, resulting in the repetition's becoming an aversive stimulus event, and c) the later punishing behavior of the parent in attempting to terminate this aversive 'nagging' behavior of the child. These relations are often seen in the development of stuttering (early positive reinforcement for child's repetitions, later punishment for child's repetitions, and negative reinforcement for parent's behavior). In this sense, the child and the parent may be conditioning one another, since each provides occasioning and reinforcing stimuli for their respective responses.

In addition to the development of repetition under such haphazard schedules of reinforcement, any one occasion for the repetition response may come under the control of other contingencies. These would include discriminative stimuli associated with different listeners, situations, and types of verbal behavior, each of which may provide a unique schedule of reinforcement that interacts with the others. The child may soon discriminate those occasions for which repeated utterances are reinforced.

A different type of contingency for the repetition response may be found in relation to aversive stimuli. It has been observed in animals and humans that initially neutral conditions, when paired with painful or unpleasant events, acquire control over the individual's behavior. Because of past experiences, the organism may respond to these stimuli as signals of undesirable things to come, and so leave the field of action (avoidance), or it may show a depression in strength of already ongoing operant behavior ("anxiety"). The complexity of the behavior produced in such situations is increased if aversive or conditioned aversive events (punishment) appear following certain behavior patterns of the organism. A child may show avoidance of certain unpleasant conditions by his verbal behavior. The repetition response may be emitted to postpone or avoid aversive conditions associated with a later portion of a verbal response. Thus, if a child is confronted with the necessity for making a verbal response which may have aversive consequences, such as those which occur in lying or in admitting his responsibility in an accident, he may be observed to postpone or avoid his response by repeating a word or a phrase prior to that crucial aversive portion of his statement.

Conversational Pauses, Interruptions, and Silence

Repetition may also arise from early training to speak in a specified pattern established in polite conversation with a listener. Children typically seem to be conditioned quite early (perhaps through a combination of mild, positive reinforcement and mild punishment) that two people in conversation do not talk at exactly the same time. There is a conversational sequence to be maintained in polite society such that first one person talks and then the other. The silence of the conversational partner may serve as the occasion for one's emission of speech, while the sound of the partner's voice can serve as the occasion for silence (and presumably listening) in oneself. Significant deviations from this pattern can result in mild punishment.

Sometimes the conversational partner's silence is only a short pause while he is composing his response, and is not meant to be the occasion for speech in the child. If the child speaks on this occasion, it is probable that the first speaker will interrupt him (perhaps irritably) and continue with the remainder of his response. This will result in the child' silence since his partner's voice has become the occasion for his silence. If this happens frequently enough, repetitions and long pauses may become a recurring pattern in the child's speech. A complex process of differential reinforcement, involving possibly both positive reinforcement and punishment, may strengthen the discriminative properties of silence in the speaking partner. It almost seems as though the child tests the situation under these circumstances in learning to discriminate whether his conversational partner's silence is or is not an occasion for his emission of speech. His partner's silence was heretofore the occasion for the child's utterance. This in turn was the occasion for his partner's silence. These events are not occurring in the accustomed sequence when the partner's silence is merely a pause and the child's utterance is the occasion for an interruption by his conversational partner.

If the speech patterns of the partner are persistently of the sort described, the child may frequently emit the first sound and wait briefly for the interruption. If the interruption is not forthcoming, he repeats the first sound as part of the originally intended message unit and continues with the remainder of his utterances. This repetition pattern in the child's speech may be maintained in great strength under such circumstances. The early conditioning of silence as an occasion for talking in a specified sequence may be quite important in dealing with the later problem of stuttering. This analysis may represent in behavioral terms what clinically is referred to as 'competition for talking time'. It seems possible to study not only the early development of repetitions in relation to alternate silent and vocal periods as discriminative stimuli, but also the reinforcing contingencies, such as punishment for deviations from this sequence and social approval and social interaction as forms of positive reinforcement.

Self-editing and Correcting

It is recognized that speakers very often 'compose' and 'edit' and 'prompt' themselves for their verbal behavior even as they are currently emitting verbal responses (*16*, pp. 255-258, 344-383). Verbal behavior is emitted in rather discrete, staccato units of varying sizes and dimensions. It is punctuated by pauses during which we assume that the processes of composition and editing go on. The speaker's emission of speech and its editing and composition are almost simultaneous activities. As he hears and feels himself talk, the speaker monitors what he hears. Occasionally he changes and corrects various aspects of his utterances such as his articulation, his pitch, his rhythm or his combination of phonemes. Such changes and corrections are expressed in the forms of short repetitions of sounds or words. Under these circumstances the speaker, as his own listener, is providing positive and negative self-reinforcements for his speech behavior. However, this composing process also may be in part under the control of the 'attending' of the listener. As long as 'attending' is forthcoming, composition and speech emission continue. When 'attending' is withdrawn, speech (and presumably composition) diminishes. It is possible that the repetition response may serve to hold this attention of the listener during composition. Therefore, it is also possible that while a child is composing his response and is making available those portions of his verbal behavior that are weak, he emits repetitions. Furthermore, such repetitions may also serve to fill the silence produced by the pauses for composition, and therefore prevent the listener from responding to those silences by speaking.

Stuttering

In transposing stuttering phenomena into the operant conditioning paradigm it is necessary to select specific stimulus patterns which should be analyzed for their functions as reinforcing conditions or as occasions for the emission of stuttering responses. It also seems necessary to define those forms of responses which shall be classed as a "stuttering response."

It is recognized that the term *stuttering* confuses rather than clarifies a behavioral analysis. It is being used here as a short-hand term in deference to its general history to designate a very general class of responses with which this analysis shall be concerned. The word "stuttering" seems to have very little utility because it is not clearly descriptive of behavior. However, it does reflect a general verbal response by a community of listeners. At present, the stuttering response, as applied to the speaker, seems to resist a precise overall definition for three basic reasons. First, the response shows variability of form from one stutterer to another, and within the same stutterer, both historically and episodically. It is quite possible that the history and longevity of a specific form of verbal behavior is the significant feature that determines whether or not it is to be classed by the clinician as stuttering. Moreover, the process of changing the form of a response (including the environmental events which constitute the occasion for such change). which can only be analyzed through its history, may be as important as any unique topographical features of a single response in cataloguing the response forms called stuttering. Perhaps there has been too great a preoccupation with the form of stuttering responses and a subordination of environmental events that are also part of the context of "stuttering" behavior. It seems premature and perhaps totally inaccurate to state that all of those forms of responses now classed as stuttering are controlled in the same way and by the same contingencies. Experimentation may well reveal several classes of responses under the control of radically different contingencies. For example, where one class of responses is controlled through negative reinforcement and another class of responses through positive reinforcement, it would be quite misleading to suggest that these responses are dynamically similar by lumping them together under one blanket term or single definition. Second, it has been observed that many forms of stuttering responses are only occasionally made public for observation. The overt verbal behavior of the stutterer which has been so aptly described recently by Bloodstein and by Johnson is an excellent beginning for such analysis. If our analysis is to be sensitive to the problem without resort to the creation of internal explanatory mechanisms, which lead us away from behavior, and therefore away from its control, we must also develop methods for making the stutterer's private (covert verbal) events accessible for observation. Analyzing the introspective verbal behavior of the stutterer just as we analyze his other overt responses may be a promising approach if the stutterer can be properly trained for such operations. Such a step would be a refinement of procedures already used clinically when stutterers are asked to report how they feel. Third, the various current theoretical explanations of stuttering employ different abstract and inferential languages and dimensions, which do not necessarily reflect the observable behavioral data. We do not have a common language for talking about stuttering. Where one person may speak of "libidinal energy," a second may speak of "anxiety-drive," a third may speak of "anticipatory-struggle," and a fourth of "situational conflict," etc. The burden of communicating among ourselves, at the technical level, in several theoretically foreign languages results in many diverse definitions of the problem. Perhaps our most useful definitions of stuttering responses will emerge from behavioral analyses based on these paradigms, if only because they demand that we retain the dimensional systems of these observations in the definitions.

Three basic propositions are offered regarding stuttering:

a) Continuities exist between nonfluency and stuttering.

b) An operant definition of stuttering should include the environmental circumstances associated with specific forms of stuttering responses and their processes of change and deterioration.

c) There is no single, simple contingency for stuttering. It is maintained by positive and negative reinforcements on complex, multiple schedules.

These propositions are contained in the discussion which follows, suggesting specific contingencies and hypotheses for study.

Continuities between Nonfluency and Stuttering

Much attention has been given to the separation of those speech responses classed as nonfluency from those classed as stuttering. If instead of these two covering terms, we employed behavioral dimensions of description, we might observe many similarities and perhaps even a continuity of the forms of these response classes as well as of their controlling contingencies. .

There may be some etiological relations between the early conditioning paradigms of nonfluency and the later conditioning paradigms that may be associated with stuttering. It is likely that conditions aversive for the child surrounding the presence of the parent during the emission of nonfluency responses will persist or even increase in strength when or if stuttering develops. By the same token, any conditions aversive for the parent concomitant with the child's nonfluency may generalize to the nonfluency and thus set the stage for a parental response which attempts to terminate the nonfluency through punishment. The parent may be conditioned to punish the child's nonfluency through negative reinforcement, since the parents' interruptions and corrections seem to terminate, momentarily, the aversive nonfluency.

The conditioning of parental responses to nonfluency may be an antecedent to parental responses associated with stuttering. The postponement of aversive consequences achieved by nonfluency repetition responses is also achieved by stuttering, perhaps in even more subtle ways. Finally, the early conditioning of silence and its functions as both a response and the occasion for a response already described for nonfluency, may have an antecedent relation to its functions in stuttering.

Contingencies for Changing Forms of Speech Responses

Studies by Johnson (*9, 10*) and by Bloodstein (*1, 2, 3*) have suggested ways in which nonfluency responses may change in form as stuttering develops. These changes in form of response reportedly occur in situations in which nonfluency is punished. The act of changing the form of the response may be the stuttering itself, made as an avoidance response. Further, their findings suggest that the auditory feedback of the vocal utterance to the stutterer has taken on aversive stimulus properties. These observations reflect not only the operant nature of stuttering behavior, but also suggest many specific variables and contingencies which should be submitted to investigation.

Paradigms and contingencies for study, which might reflect the acquisition and maintenance of stuttering responses, appear in Table 1. These paradigms may be descriptive of events which occur a number of times and in a number of settings and are only representative outlines for study. They are presented here to delineate classes of events which should be investigated. While they all suggest the descriptive contingencies which might be encountered in stuttering, the first four are suggestive of a developmental sequence.

TABLE I

REPRESENTATIVE PARADIGMS IN STUTTERING

Stimulus	Response	Consequence
1 Listener	Nonfluency	No differential reinforcement
2. Listener	Nonfluency	Punishment
3. Aversive listener (threat of punishment)	Changes nonfluency (struggle or silence)	(a) Avoids aversive stimuli of nonfluency and/or (b) Punishment for new response
4. Threatening audience	Changes response i.e., repetition to silence to prolonging, etc.	(a) Terminates ongoing aversive stimuli of punishing audience and/or (b) Punishment for new response
5. Sound of own voice (auditory feedback to stutterer)	Changes response	Terminates preceding aversive response form
6. Listener	Changes response	Positive reinforcement for changing response
7. Other S^D occasions (child may want something)	Stuttering	Positive reinforcement (gains attention) (given desired object)

Number 1, in Table 1, shows the most frequently encountered event for children who do not later develop stuttering, that is, no differential reinforcement for nonfluency. In this contingency, positive reinforcements are provided by listeners for the child's verbal behavior in general. If nonfluencies are emitted, they are usually followed by the positively reinforcing stimuli provided for the other properties of verbal behavior. The important feature is that nonfluency is not differentially reinforced as a class of responses. Nonfluency does not become a discriminative stimulus for differential listener activity. An interesting analysis would be that of tracing the decrement of nonfluency—especially when we recognize that nonfluency responses can be maintained by their connections to reinforcement schedules for other behavior. An analysis of these connections may in part reveal the dynamics of current nonfluencies commonly observed in the speech of non-stutterers.

Number 2 suggests that a child's nonfluent responses were punished. It has been suggested earlier that in studying this class of events, attention must be given to the mutual conditioning of the child and the parent—that is, the occasioning and reinforcing stimuli which control the forms of speech responses emitted by the child, and the occasioning and reinforcing stimuli which control the 'punishment' responses of a parent. This necessarily involves an historical and developmental analysis as well as an analysis of the current status of these variables.

Numbers 3 and 4 suggest that the punisher (listener) has become a conditioned aversive stimulus. As such, this listener may generate an 'emotional situation' and the child emits verbal responses (different forms of stuttering) which both terminate on-going aversive stimuli emanating from the listener (frowns and grimaces) and attempt to avoid aversive consequences of the original nonfluency response (admonitions and corrections by listener). It can be observed that the original form of the nonfluency response is changed. In fact there may be several cycles of change in response form until a dynamic equilibrium evolves in which the positive reinforcements (listener's attention and social interaction) for a particular pattern of responses are more potent than either their aversive consequences or the reinforcements for changing the response form. Thus, clinically, we see the original, effortless repetition pattern degenerate into response forms that are characterized by muscular tension, bizarre articulatory postures and movements, facial grimaces, unusual phonation and respiratory patterns, and prolonged periods of silence.

Accompanying these behaviors may be other secondary behaviors somewhat remote from the vocal mechanism, such as closing the eyes, stamping the foot, pounding the fist, or violently shaking the head. If these behaviors happened to be emitted when reinforcement was provided for the verbal response, they too may become a part of the stutterer's recurring repertoire.

Number 5 in Table 1 suggests that the stutterer is responding as his own listener to his aversive speech forms. By changing the form of his stuttering, from moment to moment, he is also terminating each preceding form. We see operating in these instances the contingencies of punishment and of negative reinforcement.

Numbers 6 and 7 suggest contingencies of positive reinforcement for maintaining stuttering. The possibility that stuttering is maintained by situations in which both positive and negative reinforcements appear has been suggested often in clinical reports. There is the feeling that the stutterer gains attention (positive reinforcement), develops an excuse for failure (negative reinforcement), and in general shifts the responsibilities for his inadequacies from himself to his stuttering and society. He has available a reason for his academic, social, and occupational failures. Williams (17) has very aptly described this shifting of responsibility by a further step. His discussion of the mystical 'it,' inside the stutterer, suggests that the stutterer is trying to relieve himself of any responsibility for emitting the undesirable behavior.

A very important, but as yet undefined, variable in these paradigms is the schedules of punishment and negative and positive reinforcements which are necessary to stabilize a stuttering response. We must know whether the stutterer's responses are reinforced each time they are emitted; whether reinforcements are provided in some uniform ratio system in terms of a given number of responses, or a given passage of time; or whether the scheduling of reinforcements is variable. Such information is important when the issues of extinction and control are considered. However, this information can become available only through appropriately de-signed studies.

Specific Occasioning, Aversive, and Reinforcing Stimuli

In a detailed analysis of stuttering, many contingencies suggest themselves as being worthy of study, e.g., "silence," both as a response and as a stimulus, "sensory feedback" to the stutterer, and specific reinforcers and models of behavior provided by the listening community.

Silence. First, there is the silence in the stutterer's audience, which can constitute an occasion for the stutterer to start talking. This would be directly related to the earlier conditioning of talking in a specified sequence. However, for a person with a past history of stuttering, the silence of the listener may also have aversive stimulus properties. The silence of the listener has sometimes been an occasion on which his speech responses were punished.

Second, there is the silence of the stutterer. As a response his silence may delay or avoid punishment by his listeners (including himself) which has occasionally followed his utterances. However, stutterers have reported that during their silences they are often quite actively engaged in various types of covert behavior. They may rehearse their response, select and reject words they cannot say, wait for the listener to begin talking again, or make an effort at articulating without phonating. Therefore, in addition to being an avoidance response by stutterers, their silence can serve as a discriminative stimulus for the emission of these covert responses. It is possible that the positive and aversive properties of the listener's silence combine with the positive and aversive properties of the stutterer's silence to provide a complex occasion for the stutterer to emit various types of responses, overt, covert, verbal and nonverbal. The result may be a complicated vacillating response, depending in part on the current deprivations operating for the stutterer and in part on the reinforcing contingencies.

The previous paragraphs attempted to describe how some properties of silent periods during conversations may apply to the problem of stuttering. We suggest that the general properties of the silent periods in conversations are no different for stutterers than they are for people with no speech problem. However, there is a difference in frequency of occurrence or magnitude of strength of these properties of silence as a function of the history of reinforcement and punishment for the stutterer.

Multiple Reinforcement of Responses to Sensory Feedback

The nexus of stimulus conditions that surround the hearing of one's own utterances is common to both stutterer and nonstutterer. Again the difference is one of frequency of occurrence and magnitude.

When a speaker emits an utterance, he responds as his own listener to many properties of the speech sounds he has emitted, e.g., the content, the tempo, the pitch, and the relations of these to the preceding conversational content. He responds also to private stimuli such as tactual-kinesthetic sensations including articulatory and breathing movements. He responds to certain public stimuli such as facial expressions of listeners, their interjected utterances, and their general postural dispositions, including eye contact.

In considering the advanced stutterer as an observer of these public and private stimuli, we may examine some typical clinical reports. One stutterer has reported, "If I pause for a comma, I'm lost," indicating he is vaguely aware that his silence is related to his stuttering, as well as some heightened sensitivities to the feedback of his utterances. Another stutterer reports that he gets a tight feeling in his throat or feels out of breath. This stutterer has indicated a response to his tactual and kinesthetic sensations in emitting his utterance. Still other stutterers have reported they cannot say the first sound of a particular word, such as their name, indicating their response to a specific stimulus and reinforcement history.

These reports indicate that such individuals have in the past been taught by the controlling community to be more sensitive to these properties. Such admonitions as "stop and start again," "think, before you talk," "take a deep breath and relax," or "if you can't say that word, say another one," are all common examples of efforts of the community to correct the condition. A by-product of such efforts is a heightening of the stutterer's awareness of these concomitants of his speech.

The pairing of these public and private stimuli with these corrective admonitions may set the stage for very complex conditioning. For example, a particular stimulus, such as a sensation of articulatory movement, may become aversive because of its connections with community admonitions. The stutterer may then emit a response (some form of stuttering) which terminates these aversive articulatory sensations, thus maintaining his stuttering through negative reinforcement.

Paradoxically, the positive reinforcements provided by the community for attending to one's articulation and breathing, for stopping and starting and repeating utterances, and for circumlocutions may also partially account for the maintenance of these behaviors in stuttering. By providing positive reinforcement for these behaviors, the community actually teaches the stutterer to stutter in certain specific ways. However, the positive reinforcements provided by listeners for each single response form may also increase the frequency of *changing the response* form as well as the frequency of emission of one particular class of response. The agents of positive reinforcement for a particular form of response may unknowingly be strengthening the behavior of shifting rapidly from one class of responses to another, thus further endangering fluency.

It is possible that the very same behaviors described above could be emitted because they terminate the aversive conditions associated with immediately preceding forms of stuttering. The stutterer may rapidly change his forms of stuttering responses (in an almost ritualistic pattern) because each succeeding response form (prolonging, repeating, silence, etc.) terminates the immediately preceding aversive form. These responses may also be emitted to terminate aversive stimuli emanating from his listener; such as "tense waiting," or "empathic mouthing" of the word.

There is the likelihood that positive reinforcement and negative reinforcement coexist in maintaining stuttering responses. The contrapuntal operation of these two reinforcement paradigms may exert a multiple control over stuttering. Their multiple strength is quite different from the controls exerted by each of these contingencies individually or in summated series. An analysis of these two different conditioning paradigms in series may reveal the variables controlling the stutterer's detailed alternation of speech responses, ie., silence, rapid repetition of first sound, silence, prolonging, etc.

Self-reinforcement

Thus far we have limited our discussion to the community as the agent of positive and negative reinforcement. However, just as a stutterer may reinforce another speaker, he may reinforce himself. We observe in the early development of speech in infants that single utterances appear sometimes to act as self-reinforcers. That is, a child may repeat sequences of similar sounds, or similar phrases or similar sentences, following the first emission. Such self-reinforcement appears to be interrupted easily. However, at a later age such self-reinforcement is more obvious. At the age of three to four years, before the child has learned to conceal his verbal behavior and while he is still playing alone, we may observe him borrowing from the parent expressions that imply positive or negative reinforcement or punishment. He may be talking aloud and using such terms as "that's a good boy," "no, no, ,you can't," "wait till Daddy comes home," or inflections which parrot adult vocal patterns. We may observe this same behavior in adults when they 'think out loud' or begin to talk to themselves during prolonged periods of isolation. We may infer from these observations that such self-reinforcement for verbal behavior goes on covertly for all speakers, including stutterers.

Because of its subtlety as a controlling variable, the covert reinforcing or aversive event is of special interest for the problem of stuttering. Quite often during clinical interviews, stutterers have been heard to report that as long as they hear themselves talking, they feel that they can go on emitting speech. Frequently their emissions of speech are short, rapid bursts of perseverative utterances which serve to "keep their motor running." Such reports suggest that stutterers reinforce themselves in emitting a chain of verbal responses. On the other hand, stutterers have reported the accumulation of "anticipations" and "dread" of stuttering and that they covertly verbalize these ideas. The result is often a long period of silence which sometimes terminates such covert verbalizing. On other occasions they emit speech "to get it over with," suggesting that their utterance terminates their aversive "anticipation."

Sometimes the stutterer's repetitions and prolongations of the first sounds of words seem to postpone or avoid more aversive forms of stuttering characterized by extreme muscular tension and silence. As the stutterer emits his verbal responses containing pauses and repetitions of fragments of words he may be: a) positively reinforced by the sound of his voice, or b) threatened by the accumulation of aversive effects of his stuttering response. The positive and negative self-reinforcing characteristics of his own voice may also exert control over his emissions of alternating forms of verbal responses.

Respondent Conditioning

Certain classes of responses that covary with stuttering are as yet poorly understood and therefore of indeterminate importance. These classes may be roughly defined as autonomic or visceral reactions such as flushing, perspiring, tremors, and changes in respiratory depth and rate. It appears that these responses can be elicited by initially neutral stimulus patterns through the process of classical conditioning. The appearance of such autonomic accompaniments to operant behavior is common in situations involving punishment or avoidance conditioning. This has been observed in both human and animal experiments. The precise relationship between operant and classical conditioning has not been defined experimentally. Skinner has implied that there is an antecedent-consequent relationship between respondent conditioning and operant conditioning such as in avoidance, escape, and punishment (*15*, pp. 160-193). It would not serve our purpose to go into the details of what is called respondent-operant overlap conditioning except to suggest that this may be one model for future investigation of the interaction of positive and negative reinforcement in maintaining stuttering.

Implications for Research on Therapy

Because these formulations are in a very early stage, and because experimentation to support these ideas has yet to be done, the application of principles of operant behavior to therapy must be approached with an attitude of skepticism. Goldiamond has already demonstrated that stuttering can be manipulated through operant conditioning techniques (*7, 8*), and that it may therefore be viewed as operant behavior under some conditions. The variables he selected to use as reinforcing and (or) discriminative stimuli seemed to be easily available for laboratory manipulation, and were directly related to the demonstrative nature of his projects.

However, clinicians have also been demonstrating the operant nature of stuttering and of their clinical transactions for some time. These "clinical demonstrations" of operant conditioning, although not based specifically on laboratory-derived principles, show a great deal of similarity to the procedures and data of the laboratory. Both the clinician and the experimenter are empirical in their attitude. Both introduce independent variables and analyze the occasions for responses. Both attempt to shape behavior and both observe relations between the stutterer's responses and consequent reactions in the stutterer's listening community. Therefore, it is felt that in addition to studies like Goldiamond's, attempts should be made to examine those variables encountered in the clinical problem of stuttering. Precisely controlled laboratory studies which are relevant (in content) to the clinical problem for the stutterer and for the clinician as reinforcing or discriminative stimuli may provide significant content for later application to therapeutic procedures. Our present knowledge about extinction of learned responses may offer some important guide lines for future laboratory research on stuttering. We know that responses acquired through variable-interval schedules of reinforcement and through avoidance conditioning seem to resist extinction. We also know that responses acquired through continuous positive reinforcement are relatively easy to extinguish. By viewing the clinical events encountered in the problem of stuttering within these paradigms and schedules of reinforcement we may find that various combinations of schedules during experimental manipulations may reveal extinction processes that have direct application to clinical management. For example, it might be possible to determine whether a response that is acquired through avoidance conditioning can be brought under the control of positive reinforcement; and in turn, whether the extinction of such a response would be easier to accomplish than the extinction of a response acquired through avoidance conditioning alone. It seems reasonable to extend the techniques for such study to include the clinical interview as a basic experimental vehicle. As such, the principles of operant behavioral analysis and manipulation can be brought closer to the problem of stuttering as it is encountered by clinician and stutterer.

Perhaps as clinicians we should immediately come to peace with ourselves as men of good will by acknowledging that all therapy is a form of controlling behavior. Recent research evidence supporting this statement has been summarized and presented by Kanfer (*11, 12*), Krasner (*13*), and Salzinger and Pisoni (*14*). It has been demonstrated that the content of verbal behavior of individuals in a variety of interview, therapeutic, and conversational situations can be controlled by the verbal responses emitted by their interviewers. Such seemingly nondirective comments as "yes" or "uh-huh" by the interviewer have been shown to be powerful reinforcing stimuli. It is no longer an issue of control versus no control by the clinician. It is now an issue of what form the controls take, whether they are valid and well founded in principle, and whether they are compatible with the ethical values of our culture.

When contingencies such as those already described have been identified in the behavior of the stutterer, we have available the raw materials for therapeutic manipulation. Such manipulations in general consist of attempts by the clinician to control the stutterer's environment. The clinician can make available to him or withhold from him those specific occasions and reinforcing contingencies which are related to the emission and extinction of his stuttering responses. In a sense, the clinician may recreate for the stutterer a small sample of his life situation in terms of controlling variables. The clinician himself becomes a part of that life situation by becoming the chief source of occasions and reinforcements for speech. The scope of this controlled environment cannot now be defined.

It is possible that experimentation on this particular topic may reveal the efficacy of total control and reconditioning in an isolated environment where all variables are systematically introduced. The technique of removing the stutterer from the complexities of a punishing society for purposes of gradual reconditioning is not too different from those procedures employed in hospitalizing patients with medical and psychiatric disorders. The advantages and disadvantages of such a technique, of course, remain to be determined through research.

The clinician has available discriminative stimuli and reinforcing stimuli only to the extent that his analysis of the history and current behavior of the stutterer is both accurate and exhaustive. Such analysis must include the practices of those members of the community who commonly reinforce the stutterer's speech behavior, e.g., parents, friends, teachers. These reinforcing practices of listeners (including the stutterer) must not be regarded as fixed controlling techniques. They are behavior patterns that have been acquired and that may therefore be amenable to re-education also. We must determine how the responses of these listeners are acquired and maintained, and how they can be modified. One major issue here is whether our direct modifications of the stutterer's forms of stuttering have any effect on the listener's reinforcing practices. In many cases, the clinician may find it more profitable to deal with the stutterer's listening community than with the stutterer.

If we retain the viewpoint that the behavior of the stutterer represents only a part of the total set of transactions between him and his community, and if we can identify the functions of the community (including clinicians) in these transactions our experimental analyses will contribute to the understanding of social behavior as well as to the problem of stuttering.

Summary

Nonfluency and stuttering are examined in the framework of operant conditioning. Relations are hypothesized between repetitions in speech and the following variables:

a. Listeners' "attending" behavior.
b. Coincidental reinforcements for other behavior.
c. States of deprivation.
d. Avoidance of aversive stimuli.
e. Conversational pauses, interruptions, and silence.
f. Self-editing and correcting.

With regard to stuttering the following propositions are offered:

a. A continuity exists between stuttering and nonfluency.

b. An operant definition of stuttering includes the stimulus and reinforcement history of specific forms of responses.

c. Stuttering is maintained by positive and negative reinforcements on complex, multiple schedules.

Events relevant to stuttering include:

a. Antecedent conditioning during nonfluency.

b. Aversive stimuli from listeners.

c. Changes in the form of stuttering.

d. "Silence" as a stimulus and as a response.

e. Sensory feedback to the stutterer.

f. Reinforcers and models of behavior provided by the community.

The clinical interview may provide an opportunity for experiments in operant conditioning to test these interpretations of stuttering.

References

Bloodstein, O.: The development of stuttering: I. Changes in nine basic features. *J. Speech Hearing Dis., 25:* 219-237, 1960.

Bloodstein, O.: The development of stuttering: II. Developmental phases. *J. Speech Hearing Dis., 25*: 366-376, 1960.

Bloodstein, O.: The development of stuttering: III. Theoretical and clinical implications. *J. Speech Hearing Dis., 26*: 67-82, 1961.

Davis, Dorothy M.: The relation of repetitions in the speech of young children to certain measures of language maturity and situational factors. Part I. *J. Speech Dis., 4*: 303-318, 1939.

Davis, Dorothy M.: The relation of repetitions in the speech of young children to certain measures of language maturity and situational factors. Part II. *J. Speech Dis., 5:* 235-241, 1940.

Davis, Dorothy M.: The relation of repetitions in the speech of young children to certain measures of language maturity and situational factors. Part III. *J. Speech Dis., 5*: 242-246, 1940.

Goldiamond, I.: Blocked speech communication and delayed feedback: An experimental design. Technical Report No. 1, Progress Report, February, 1960. Operational Applications Laboratory, Air Force Cambridge Research Center, Bedford, Massachusetts.

Goldiamond, I.: The temporal development of fluent and blocked speech communication. Final Report and Technical Report Nos. 2, 3, & 4, September, 1960. Operational Applications Laboratory, Air Force Cambridge Research Center, Bedford, Massachusetts.

Johnson, W.: The role of evaluation in stuttering behavior. *J. Speech Dis., 3:* 85-89, 1938.

Johnson, W.: A study of the onset and development of stuttering. *J. Speech Dis., 7:* 251-257, 1942.

Kanfer, F. H.: Verbal rate, content, and adjustment ratings in experimentally structured interviews. *J. Abnorm. Soc. Psychol., 58:* 305-311, 1959.

Kanfer, F., Phillips, J., Matarazzo, J. and Saslow, G.: Experimental modification of interviewer content in standardized interviews. *J. Consule. Psychol., 24:* 528-536, 1960.

Krasner, L.: Studies of the conditioning of verbal behavior. *Psychol. Bull., 55:* 148-170, 1958.

Salzinger, K. and Pisoni, S.: Reinforcement of verbal affect responses of normal subjects during the interview. *J. Abnorm. Soc. Psychol., 60:* 127-130, 1960.

Skinner, B. F.: *Science and Human Behavior.* New York, Macmillan, 1953.

Skinner, B. F.: *Verbal Behavior.* New York, Appleton-Century-Crofts, Inc., 1957.

Williams, D. E.: A point of view about 'Stuttering.' *J. Speech Hearing Dis., 22:* 390-397, 1957.

Winitz, H.: Repetitions in the vocalizations and speech of children in the first two years of life. *J. Speech Hearing Dis., Monog. Supplement No. 7:* 55-62, 1951.

5

An Inquiry into the Use of Inter-personal Communication as a Source for Therapy with Stutterers

Eugene B. Cooper, Ed.D.

Introduction

The observation that stutterers experience difficulties in inter-personal relationships is not a new one. Most authorities on stuttering have discussed the stutterer's difficulties in inter-personal relationships. Diehl (6), for example, recently noted that there is a sufficient body of evidence to conclude that the stutterer's emotional disturbances and adjustment problems are rooted in his poor inter-personal relationships.

At the same time, most authorities on stuttering therapy note that the inter-personal relationship between the therapist and the stutterer is perhaps the most important single factor in therapeutic success. Murphy and FitzSimons, for example, stated that:

> Much of the past therapeutic success of speech clinicians with stutterers can be attributed to the undefined emotional relationship that existed between clinician and stutterer, rather than to the specific speech-correction technique employed (9, p. 8).

Despite the acknowledgement that the therapeutic relationship is of primary importance to the therapeutic success, there have been few discussions in the literature regarding stuttering therapy which attempt to define or indicate the nature of a good therapeutic relationship. Bloodstein, in discussing the importance of the therapeutic relationship, noted this failure to define the therapeutic relationship: "This relationship may be either left to chance or deliberately molded to conform to a specific conception of what it should be like. Too frequently it is merely allowed to develop as it will" (3, p. 52).

Martin, while noting the importance of the interaction between client and therapist, observed the need for defining the relationship. He stated that we should view speech therapy as a process ". . . occurring in an inter-personal relationship and operating on principles or laws to be discovered or further explored" (8, p. 578).

Diehl (6) has noted the difficulties in successfully utilizing the Rogerian Client Centered approach with stutterers. He observed that the therapist is encouraged to direct the stutterer in overcoming certain symptomatic habit patterns and at the same time to be accepting and permissive with the client in order to develop a meaningful inter-personal relationship. Diehl observed that such a "chameleon-like relationship" would undoubtedly dangerously confuse and bewilder the client, and even, perhaps, develop in the client serious symptoms of anxiety.

Diehl, in noting his agreement with Barbara (2) as to the type of client-therapist relationship which best meets the needs of stutterers, observed that:

> . . . from the beginning the therapist must present a firm, consistent, objective attitude. Such an attitude need not, of course, be displayed with brutal disregard for any suffering the patient may be experiencing. Firmness and consistency should not be confused by the therapist with pompous arrogance and defensive dogmatism. Firmness and consistency are not incompatible with kindness and warmth in relating to others (6, p. 151).

Important similarities between the therapeutic relationship in stuttering therapy and the therapeutic relationship in psychotherapy have been noted. Bloodstein, for example, stated: "In the author's opinion there is one kind of relationship which is far more suitable for the stuttering therapy situation than any other, and that is what might appropriately be termed a clinical relationship" (3, p. 52).

Sheehan, in noting the importance of the therapeutic relationship in stuttering observed that: "The stutterer who is able to perceive what speech therapy offers undergoes a profound psychotherapeutic experience" (11, p. 478).

Cooper (5), after investigating the inter-relationships among client progress in stuttering therapy, the nature of the affect interchange between client and therapist, and certain personality characteristics of both client and therapist, concluded that his findings constituted the first "research" support for observations that important similarities exist between stuttering therapy and psychotherapy.

In psychotherapy, as in stuttering therapy, the relationship between client and therapist is generally acknowledged as being the single most important factor in therapeutic success. Despite this, views of the psychotherapeutic relationship have generally been pragmatic conclusions based upon extensive clinical experience, and have not been subjected to measurement (13)

Recently, Snyder defined the therapeutic relationship:

> . . . as a reciprocity of various sets of affective attitudes which two or more persons hold toward each other in psychotherapy . . . . Thus the relationship must consist . . . of some sort of mathematical relation between transference and countertransference attitudes (13, p. 270).

Following an extensive research program aimed at defining and quantifying important affective attitudes in the relationship, Snyder concluded that the relationship could be dealt with in measurable terms.

In view of the observed importance of the therapeutic relationship in stuttering therapy, and because a therapeutic relationship can now be discussed in more meaningful (and presumably measurable) terms, a system of stuttering therapy which relies on the therapeutic relationship for its "cornerstone" appears relevant and appropriate. Inter-Personal Communications Therapy (IPC Therapy) is based on the concept that through the therapist's control and manipulation of the therapeutic relationship, the stutterer undergoes a meaningful learning experience in inter-personal relationships which enables him to modify that behavior resulting from distorted perceptions of inter-personal relationships.

Assumptions and Principles

Any system of therapy must necessarily be founded on assumptions regarding the nature of the problem being treated and the nature of the therapeutic techniques being employed. IPC Therapy has been constructed upon the following set of assumptions regarding the nature of stuttering and the nature of the therapeutic experience:

A. *Stutterers, like other persons, strive for self-actualization and have the capacity and motivation to achieve wholeness.*

This is a restatement of a basic tenet of Roger's (10) Client Centered Therapy. While discussing therapy for stutterers, Bloodstein observed: "All good therapy is based upon a belief in the individual's innate capacity for emotional growth" (3, p. 52).

B. *Stuttering is a learned response indicative of a maladaptive reaction to inter-personal relationships.*

IPC Therapy was created on the assumption that stuttering, as Murphy and FitzSimons have noted:

> . . . is a learned, nonintegrative, self-defensive reaction to anxiety or fear of threatening circumstances with which the person feels incapable of coping . . . the *roots* of stuttering originate in inter-personal relationships, most specifically around *verbal or nonverbal* developmental tasks during early socialization experiences with important elders" (9, p. 145).

C. *Stuttering is self-maintaining because of the continued and reinforced disruption in inter-personal relationships.*

Diehl (6) recently observed that regardless of what etiological bias the therapist has — physiological, psychological, or eclectic — the fact remains that the stutterer experiences his peculiar distress when speaking with people. Murphy and FitzSimons (9) concluded that stuttering persists primarily as a consequence of old and contemporary inter-personal discomforts.

D. *The therapeutic relationship provides a situation that can be a controlled learning experience for the stutterer in inter-personal relationships.*

Inter-personal relationships occurring outside the therapy situation often lack immediacy when discussed during therapy. Discussions of extra-therapy relationships may, in fact, encourage the stutterer to intellectualize about his problems in inter-personal relationships rather than to gain an emotional understanding of them. Also, the therapist experiences difficulties in understanding the motivations of the other person involved in the stutterer's inter-personal interaction. Thus, it is frequently difficult for the therapist to grasp the reality of the inter-personal situation the stutterer discusses in therapy. Without an understanding of the reality of the interaction, the therapist is handicapped in observing whether the stutterer's perceptions are accurate. On the other hand, the therapist is in a position to perceive more accurately the inter-action in the immediate therapeutic relationship and can therefore assist the stutterer in evaluating accurately the dynamics of the inter-action. Sheehan (11) noted that one of the therapist's chief functions is that of supplying the stutterer with the kind of relationship which he has lacked.

E. *The therapeutic relationship provides the stutterer with an inter-personal involvement which is directed by the therapist in such a manner as to facilitate the client's realistic perception of self and others in inter-personal relationships.*

Murphy and FitzSimons noted that therapy, to be successful, must assist the stutterer: ". . . to make an adequate (realistic and developmental) perception and reaction to self and surroundings (others) at the same time" (9, p. 14).

In order to accomplish the goal of aiding the stutterer to perceive himself and others more accurately, IPC Therapy emphasizes the *immediate* relationship as being the important subject for therapeutic discussion. Bandura (1) noted that clients, with the intention of rewarding the therapist as well as avoiding unpleasant topics, will discuss interesting historical material and thereby avoid the discussion of their current inter-personal problems. As Sheehan (11) observed, a most important avenue in assisting the stutterer to re-evaluate his perception of his inter-personal relationships is through an evaluation of the therapeutic relationship. Diehl (6) observed that any intrapsychical changes which occur in therapy are a direct consequence of the stutterer's more satisfying inter-personal experiences.

F. *The therapeutic relationship, by serving as a learning experience in inter-personal relationships, is of primary import-*

ance in bringing about behavioral change on the part of the stutterer.

Assuming that stuttering, as Murphy and FitzSimons (9) suggested, is the most effective behavior possible for the individual at a given moment relative to his perception of himself and others, treatment need not dwell on the forces exerted upon the individual in the past. Combs and Snygg stated:

> The emphases of perceptual psychology upon an immediate rather than a historical understanding of the causation of behavior has important implications for treatment . . . If it is true . . . that behavior is a function of perception, then it should be possible to assist people to better adjustment by helping them change their perceptions even if the counselor has no knowledge of the past. If perception can be changed, behavior must also change (4, p. 426).

IPC Therapy is based on the assumption that as the stutterer begins to perceive himself and others more accurately as a result of an effective therapeutic relationship, the stutterer becomes capable of modifying the stuttering behavior.

G. *A meaningful inter-personal relationship is an ongoing, ever changing phenomenon, which must be described in terms of its dynamic nature.*

Observations of inter-personal relationships reveal that relationships whose affective qualities do not change or fluctuate are relatively superficial. For example, a person's affective attitudes toward a colleague who is seen every day and with whom pleasantries are exchanged, but who is not directly involved in the person's social or professional life, probably remains relatively stable. In this situation, neither party is more than superficially involved in the relationship, and little or no emotional affect exists between the two. Such a relationship could be termed "friendly," "cordial," but certainly not "clinical" and not one in which behavior modification of either party would be motivated or facilitated by shifts in the affective attitudes. On the other hand, the changing nature of affective attitudes is obvious in such an emotionally significant interaction as a parent-child relationship.

The changing nature of the affective attitude held by the therapist toward the client as well as the client toward the therapist in psycho-therapy has been observed in research work such as that reported by Snyder (13). In psychotherapeutic language, this changing affect has been discussed in terms of fluctuating transference and counter-transference. Cooper (5) has presented research evidence in stuttering therapy to suggest the importance of noting the changes in affective attitudes of both the therapist and the patient in the stuttering therapy situation. Cooper concluded that it is more accurate to note stages in the therapeutic relationship than to characterize the relationship as if it were the same throughout therapy.

It is apparent that a therapist's attempt to maintain a "serene" or "homeostatic" atmosphere in the therapeutic situation is questionable. It is also apparent that the standard adjectives generally applied in the description of good therapeutic relationships (such as "warm," "friendly," "sincere," etc.) do not: 1) indicate the dynamic and ever-changing nature of a therapeutic relationship, 2) provide therapists with an understanding of how the changing nature of a therapeutic relationship can facilitate and motivate behavioral modification.

H. *The overt behavior of the stutterer (in terms of stuttering symptoms) provides the therapist with concrete behavior to manipulate, facilitating the development of a relationship process conducive to learning in the area of inter-personal relationships.*

Initially IPC Therapy is structured for the stutterer on the basis of the behavioral manifestations of the stuttering symptoms. The stuttering symptoms provide the therapist with a "handle" to lead the stutterer to an evaluation of the feelings and attitudes which influence the stuttering behavior. Van Riper (14) noted that therapy can be structured on the basis of the symptomatology and that the stutterer can be directed to modify these behaviorisms through situational assignments (e.g., directing the stutterer to control facial grimaces in varying speaking situations). Van Riper noted that such assignments are of value only when they ". . . provoke the resistance and testings of the relationship between stutterer and therapist which, when worked through, create new insights and energies for healing" (14, p. 389).

Sheehan, in noting that the symptomatology can be used to

facilitate the stutterer's examination of attitudes and feelings, observed:

> If we are really justified in viewing stuttering as an externalized conflict, should we not avail ourselves of this ready avenue to other levels? Conflict at the relationship level, for example, is mediated through situation and word fear; why not then begin where the stuttering occurs and work back to the stutterer's relationships? . . . The stutterer's blocks and his reactions to them mirror his self-concept, attitudes toward others, mechanisms for handling conflicts, and many other aspects of his personality (11, p. 148).

The Process of Therapy

In order to discuss a phenomenon whose nature changes over a period of time, it is convenient to view the nature of the phenomenon at various time intervals. Thus, IPC Therapy is presented as a process having four stages. While it will become obvious that important characteristics of one stage will also typify other stages, IPC Therapy's primary factor (the inter-personal relationship between therapist and client) is qualitatively different in each stage. That is, the four stages in IPC Therapy are each primarily dependent on varying affective attitudes which the stutterer holds toward the therapist. The stages in IPC Therapy, however, are named to suggest the therapeutic activity which leads to varying affective attitudes.

IPC Therapy requires the therapist to manipulate the therapeutic relationship through these four stages:

I. Diagnostic and Structuring Stage.
II. Examination and Confrontation Stage.
III. Introspective and Testing Stage.
IV. Symptom Modification Stage.

I. Diagnostic and Structuring Stage

As suggested by the name of this stage, the therapist is primarily concerned with achieving two goals: 1) the therapist assists the stutterer to identify those behavorial traits (i.e., all avoidance behavior such as refusal to use the telephone, and habitual overt struggle behavior such as facial contortions) which provide obvious indications of the stuttering problem: 2) the therapist indicates the procedures which can be followed to: a) remove all habitual struggle behavior and b) achieve desensitization to situations provoking avoidance reactions.

Because stutterers just entering therapy frequently are unable to objectively view or conceptualize the problem of stuttering, they typically describe their stuttering problem in terms which indicate a vague and general anxiety. It is perhaps analogous to a person who knows he is ill, but is unable to define his problem. He will live in abject fear, dreading the worst, until the illness has been diagnosed. Even if the diagnosis is a threatening one, the person generally experiences an immediate reduction of anxiety as he mobilizes his forces to face the problem or to begin actively striving for health. So it appears with stutterers. They are well aware that "something is wrong," but have been unable to grasp the exact nature of the problem and have avoided seeking a diagnosis for fear of learning something even more fearful about themselves. The therapist, in the initial meetings, leads the stutterer to identify that overt behavior which actually *is* the problem. The stutterer learns that the problem of stuttering is one of "non-fluencies," or sound repetitions, prolongations, or hesitations, which have become surrounded by many behaviorisms directed at avoiding these non-fluencies.

A method which has proven most satisfactory in aiding both the therapist and the client to identify and conceptualize the stuttering problem, has been the use of the "stuttering apple." The "stuttering apple" is created in the following manner: the therapist suggests to the stutterer that the core of his problem is the non-fluency or the "getting stuck on a word." Most stutterers readily agree that this is the *basic* problem and acknowledge that their stuttering probably began with simple non-fluency. This is drawn on a paper as a small circle and labeled either "non-fluency," "block," or simply "getting stuck." The therapist encourages the stutterer to note "things I do because I stutter, and things I do when I get stuck." As the stutterer, (frequently with suggestions by the therapist) notes such beavior as "I blink my eyes when I stutter," "My hand jerks when I get stuck," "I don't answer the phone," "I never order coffee because I always get stuck on the K sound," etc., the therapist draws a small circle attached to and surrounding the "core," writing in each circle that behavior which the stutterer has noted.

This procedure is continued until the stutterer, with the aid of the therapist, has put in the graphic display all those behaviorisms associated with the moment of stuttering (or block). Frequently, stutterer and therapist observe more client behaviorisms as therapy progresses and these are added to the graphic display. It is explained to the stutterer that a circle can be drawn around the "core" and all the attached labeled behaviorisms, and a stem added to produce the "stuttering apple." (This device was originally used with children, but it has been found to be applicable to adults as well. They do not react to what might appear as a childish manner of conceptualizing the problem.) This completed stuttering apple represents the stuttering problem on the behavioral level.

The use of the stuttering apple has thus achieved the goal of conceptualizing the client's problem on the behavioral level. The most important aspect of this manner of defining and identifying the problem is that it does not threaten the stutterer at this early stage of therapy by forcing his attention to feelings and attitudes. The same goal is achieved by focusing on behavior. That is, the client's attitudes and feelings are reflected in the behaviorisms which comprise the stuttering problem.

The therapist suggests to the stutterer that this model represents that behavior which the stutterer wants to modify or eliminate. Therapy then, will become a matter of "eating the apple to its core." The therapist can suggest that the "core" will disintegrate because the behaviorisms no longer reinforce it. The therapist can draw the "vicious cycle" of stuttering and point out to the client that, as he well knows, the harder he tries not to stutter, the more he avoids the more anxious he becomes, and consequently, the more he stutterers. The therapist suggests that the behaviorisms noted in the stuttering apple are actually attempts to avoid stuttering. Consequently, if the stutterer eliminates all of those behaviorisms, the stuttering (or core) will disintegrate.

This presentation by the therapist (in conjunction with the information regarding behavior supplied by the stutterer) has provided diagnostic information regarding the behavior of the client (and indirectly — the feelings and attitudes of the stutterer). The stuttering apple now provides the therapist and client with a graphic display of how therapy will proceed. The client usually volunteers, at this point, that therapy will be directed at taking "bites out of the apple." Now it is simply a matter of determining which behaviorism should be eliminated first. In discussion with the client, a decision is made as to which "bite" to take first. Typically the therapist leads the stutterer to choose a relatively "easy" behaviorism to eliminate such as "I blink my eyes when I stutter."

Purposely, the language of the therapist is kept at a "non-professional jargon" level. Diehl has noted that occasionally the therapist will deliberately use four syllable words in order to impress the patient with his erudition, and in fact, may gear his entire manner of speaking to demonstrate how all-knowing he is. Diehl noted:

> A relationship rooted in such an atmosphere may flourish for a short period while the patient waits for the impressive words and manner to purge him vicariously; however, when this is not forthcoming the relationship is doomed to failure (6, p. 157).

Because the therapist to this point in therapy has assisted the stutterer in visualizing and defining his stuttering problem and has not yet sought modification of that behavior by the stutterer, the client typically is positive in his affect toward the therapist. Also, the therapist has indicated specific activities to be undertaken in a prescribed fashion (through the use of the stuttering apple) aimed at modifying the stuttering behavior. The stutterer feels that the way has been made clear and is eager to begin. (How frequently we have left the doctor's office with diet in hand, consumed with eagerness to begin and blessing the good Doctor for this sense of direction — how frequently we've crept back to "that damned Doctor" to hear his threats of our own extinction for our lack of perseverance).

It is important that the stutterer experience the initial positive feelings towards the therapist because, as the next stage commences and proceeds, there must be sufficient residual positive affect on the part of the client toward the therapist to sustain the relationship. If the client does not experience positive transference to the therapist at this stage, when the therapist begins pressing the client for symptom modification in the next stage, the client may withdraw from therapy.

II. *Examination and Confrontation Stage*

In the Examination and Confrontation Stage of IPC Therapy, the therapist begins to press the stutterer for symptom modification. Having identified, during the Diagnostic and Structuring Stage, those behaviorisms associated with the stuttering problem, the therapist now requests the stutterer to begin modifying those behaviorisms. These assignments are similar to those suggested by Van Riper (14). For example, the stutterer is directed to modify his avoidance of the telephone by making a specified number of telephone calls.

Assignments such as these produce negative or resistive reactions on the part of the stutterer toward the therapist and the therapy situation. Bloodstein observed this. He stated:

> . . . such behavior is exactly what we should expect when we ask the stutterer to do so many things which he has been trying so hard for so long not to do. It is not the fact of resistance which should concern us but the form the resistance takes (3, p. 55).

Bloodstein (3) suggested three major forms that this resistance to therapy might take. He noted that the stutterer (although not consciously aware that he is resisting): 1) denies the existence of the problem; 2) openly states that he is incapable of doing anything about it, or 3) begins to intellectualize about the problem.

As in our analogy with the doctor and his diet, we find that it is not so easy to modify our eating behavior as it appeared when the doctor first laid out the procedure to be followed. Aren't we disenchanted when we find that we have to deny ourselves food; that *we* have to *do* the unpleasant task of rejecting a piece of pie. How nice it is to find that we really don't want to lose weight because then we would have to have our clothes altered, and we can't afford *that*. And then, the physician admonishes us for our lack of perseverance! So it is with stutterers. It might be concluded that the frequently noted observation of many therapists dealing with stutterers that "stutterers are hostile" is the result of this disenchantment.

IPC Therapy attempts to utilize these forms of resistance to develop a meaningful inter-personal relationship between the stutterer and the thearapist. Although the therapist is aware of resistance behavior on the part of the client, the therapist continues to press the stutterer for symptom modification. The client, unaware of his resistance, is unsuccessful in carrying out the assignments and achieving their immediate goals. Thus, during the Examination phase of the second stage in therapy, it is the therapist who is doing the examining. Through observation of the stutterer's behavior, the therapist is able to perceive the nature of the client's defense mechanisms and avoidance techniques. In effect, the therapist encourages the stutterer to express all of his defense mechanisms openly. This means that the therapist must accept these defenses and, in fact, encourage the stutterer to demonstrate his creativity in bringing about new methods of denial and defense. When the therapist feels that he has an understanding of the stutterer's mode of behavior, and is capable of grasping the dynamics underlying the client's resistance to therapy, the *Confrontation* phase of the second stage of therapy commences.

Before the therapist commences to confront the stutterer with the stutterer's resistive behavior, the therapist should be aware of the distinction between accepting a *person* and accepting *behavior*. Martin (8), made the distinction that what is accepted is the stutterer as a person, not necessarily his behavior. Sheehan stated:

> . . . the speech therapist can be permissive on the feeling level but cannot be completely permissive on the doing level, unless he is willing to work for an indefinite period in an entirely supportive (and dubiously supportive) role (11, p. 162).

Initially the therapist cites behavior, free of value judgments (in terms of the behavior being "bad" or "good"). Typically, the stutterer does not initially perceive the discrimination between acceptance as a person and rejection of his behavior. The stutterer perceives this confrontation as an indication of disapproval and rejection (to continue the analogy to dieting: when our spouse cites our behavior—taking that extra helping of potatoes—don't we feel disapproval and rejection?). It is only as the relationship continues that the stutterer is able to make the distinction that even though his avoidance behavior is cited and in essence rejected, the therapist is understanding of the feelings and attitudes which initiated such behavior.

As the therapist continues to confront the client with the observed resistive behavior, the client typically responds in a defensive manner, denying his resistive behavior or indicating intellectual acceptance of the therapist's perceptions. With continued pressuring by the therapist, signs of covert hostility begin to appear. For example, the client may become non-verbal, appear late for therapy, and subtly indicate that he feels therapy is a waste of time. These displays of covert hostility indicate that the therapist has succeeded in forcing the client to become emotionally involved in the therapeutic relationship. In other words, the therapist confronts the stutterer with the resistance behavior to force an emotional involvement on the part of the stutterer in the therapeutic situation.

The manner in which this confrontation is conducted by the therapist is crucial to the success of IPC Therapy. This requires a sensitivity on the part of the therapist as to when and how to confront the stutterer to provoke an emotional involvement in the situation without forcing the client to withdraw from the therapeutic situation. When it becomes apparent that the stutterer is emotionally involved in the therapeutic relationship, the therapist encourages him to verbalize his feelings toward the therapist.

During the time the therapist is "pushing" the client to express his honest feelings toward the therapist, the client will almost invariably ask what the therapist "wants." When this question arises, the therapist states that he is seeking a relationship in which the client can be *honest* not only with the therapist but with himself. The therapist indicates that the client *must* have "feelings" about the therapist and before the relationship can proceed meaningfully these feelings must be acknowledged. Initially the client may deny such feelings. The therapist must usually repeat this procedure for several sessions before the client feels free enough to verbalize any feelings of hostility toward the therapist.

The client may begin to express tentative indications of distress by observing that he has "felt" that therapy has become "somewhat a waste of time," or that he can't understand how his "feelings" have anything to do with his stuttering. The therapist must usually take the lead in suggesting that the client feels the therapist is probably "well meaning,' but also probably a "quack." This does not mean to imply that stutterers are any different from others in terms of their reactions to persons pressing for modification of behavior. When our doctor continually points out our lack of control on a diet, and suggests that we begin to evaluate ourselves to determine "why" we are not following the prescription, isn't the "normal" reaction one of questioning the doctor's competence and ability?

As the therapist continues to encourage the stutterer for a more direct expression of feeling toward the therapist, the client's overt verbalizations of hostility frequently reach a climax in a "torrent of negativism." In a true sense the client has "let himself go." He has "blasted" the therapist. He has openly expressed feelings which were previously held back because "it is not nice to say such things." A fairly accurate statement regarding the client's feelings up to this point in therapy might be this: "If I *really* told him how I felt, he (the therapist) would tell me to go to hell." Now the client has "told it all." The client has held back nothing of himself and is consequently without defenses. "This is the way I am—the way I feel."

When the therapist accepts and indicates understanding of the feelings expressed by the client, the client begins to introspect and say, in essence: "Why *do* I feel this way about you?" The client has begun to introspect in an environment conducive to self-examination. The client has been honest in this expression of feelings. The therapist has rewarded the expression of honest feelings by accepting the stutterer's feelings. The stutterer has undergone a learning experience, and now finds that he can express his feelings openly in an atmosphere of acceptance. In this atmosphere, the client finds he can express himself freely and can examine just why he feels as he does. This is not an intellectual process, but an emotional one.

This stage of IPC Therapy has been the most difficult stage for naive therapists (in terms of IPC Therapy) to follow. Frequently they report that as they "needle" their clients (by citing in an honest fashion the behavior they observe) they experience feelings of guilt and fear concerning their therapeutic behavior. Indeed, the therapist may report that he "feels like a sadist." As the therapist continues to openly and honestly confront the stutterer with the stutterer's own behavior, and as the stutterer's affect becomes more and more negative, the naive therapist may withdraw from the situation. The therapist finds that such confrontation is threatening not only to the client, but to himself.

It is at this point that the therapist is required to examine his own perceptions. In fact, assuming that the therapist is a perceptive and sensitive individual, he continually questions himself as to his own feelings and attitudes in the situation. The importance of the adjustment of the therapist using IPC Therapy is discussed in greater detail in the Implications portion of this chapter.

Experience has indicated that those therapists who acknowledge a commonality with their clients are those therapists who are capable of conveying a basic feeling of respect and acceptance to their clients, even while confronting them with their resistive behavior. Murphy and Fitzsimons stated:

> One of the most valuable decisions which clinicians can make is to admit their commonality with the persons whom they are trying to help . . . The principle of being different in degree and not in kind applies to all clinicians, all stutterers, all people (9, p. 104).

One means of facilitating the open expression of feeling on the part of the stutterer is that of having the therapist express *his* feelings toward the client. Because the therapist recognizes that the resistance of the client is actually the stutterer's problem and not just the stutterer's malicious intent to avoid facing himself, the therapist accepts the stutterer as a person. At the same time, therapists, being human, undoubtedly experience frustration and anger with the client for his continued dodging of the real issue: feelings. The therapist expresses these feelings of frustration to the client. The therapist is honest in his expression of feeling toward the client. This expression of feeling on the part of the therapist is, of course, selective. What is important is that the therapist be honest in *this* relationship — it does not mean that the therapist should transfer his frustrations with all his (therapist) inter-personal relationships onto the client. The therapist's expression of feeling must be accurate and justifiable in relation to the *immediate* inter-personal interaction.

The expression of feeling by the therapist regarding the immediate inter-personal interaction serves a distinct purpose in the Confrontation phase: the therapist, by his behavior, reassures the client that he (the therapist) is himself involved in the relationship and "cares about what happens." Frequently, this expression of feeling on the part of the therapist facilitates the verbalization of feeling on the part of the client.

Again, it cannot be over-stated that the therapist must have enough understanding of his own feelings regarding the relationship that his expression of feeling toward the client is warranted by the interaction taking place in the *immediate* relationship, and that the expression of feeling is to serve in developing an affective "honest" relationship. It is not atypical to hear a beginning therapist state: "I get so damned frustrated with —————, all he does is intellectualize!" The therapist is asked: "Well, did you tell him so?"

During the Examination and Confrontation Stage, the therapist, by pressuring the stutterer for symptom modification, has forced the client into an emotionally honest inter-personal relationship in which the stutterer will be able to accurately evaluate his attitudes and feelings toward himself and others.

III. Introspective and Testing Stage

Through focusing attention on overt behavior, the therapist has brought the stutterer to an emotional involvement in the therapeutic relationship. The therapist has forced the stutterer to express openly feelings of hostility toward the therapist which were accepted by the therapist who rewarded the expression of feelings (not necessarily the content of the feeling). In such a situation where one finds one's "honest" feelings are accepted, introspection is facilitated. The stutterer has found in the relationship that he is accepted — that his feelings are accepted, and he is comfortable enough in the relationship to look inward and to evaluate his feelings and perceptions. Therapy has now progressed to the third stage. The stutterer's defenses have been overcome in the therapeutic relationship and the stutterer has found he is accepted as a person on an affective level. Thus an important interpersonal learning experience for the stutterer has taken place.

During the third stage, the stutterer may "test" the therapeutic relationship. Typically this is done by covert expressions of hostility toward the therapist (i.e., absence from therapy, rejection of the therapist's evaluation of situations, etc.). The therapist confronts the stutterer with this behavior, and the "air is cleared" again by expression of feeling on the stutterer. Each of these experiences reinforces the stutterer's learning experience in an affective interpersonal relationship.

Therapists utilizing IPC Therapy have observed that it is difficult for them to shift their behavior from the preceeding stage of therapy. In that stage, they were *directive* in the sense that they pointed out to the stutterer his behavior. In this stage, as the client begins to introspect, therapists note that they have a tendency to be *directive* in the same manner as in the Examination and Confrontation Stage. This should be avoided. If the therapist continues to be directive at this point in therapy, the client may be unable to introspect freely. Frequently the therapist can see what the client cannot see and the therapist's urge to convey this insight to the client is strong. If this is done, however, the insight may be "intellectual" and may not be grasped meaningfully by the client. It is during this stage that the therapist using IPC Therapy behaves in a similar fashion to therapists utilizing the Client-Centered System of therapy as described by Rogers (10).

Generalization of learning from the therapeutic relationship to outside situations soon becomes apparent The stutterer now finds he is capable of expressing his feelings openly in other situations. Frequently, a problem in over-generalization of learning is encountered and the stutterer expresses feelings inappropriately in outside situations. Quickly, however, the client learns to discriminate when expression of feeling is appropriate and when it is not. The continuation of the affective relationship in the therapeutic situation is important for the stutterer during this "testing" stage. The rejection the client receives outside of the therapeutic situation tends to suppress expressions of affect during this period of "discriminative learning" and the client-therapist relationship provides an atmosphere in which the stutterer can evaluate and perceive these rejections accurately.

Whereas the therapy sessions during the Examination and Confrontation Stage were rather consistently intense in terms of the interaction between therapist and client, the therapist now finds that the stutterer desires and needs relatively "easy" sessions. After the Introspection phase has proceeded for several sessions the stutterer may indicate that he "just wants to chat" during a few of these sessions. At these times, the client usually is extremely verbal about rather superficial things. For example, the stutterer may indicate a desire to discuss his interest in fishing with the therapist. It is important for the therapist to recognize what the stutterer is doing and to allow this superficial interaction to take place infrequently. These "chatting" sessions are important during the Introspection and Testing Stage. Up to this time in therapy, the therapist has provided the stutterer with immediate feedback. That is, the therapist structured the therapy process in the initial stage and then began to react to the stutterer's behavior during the second stage of therapy. The stutterer was able to observe directly the manner in which his behavior was being accepted. During this third stage of therapy, however, the therapist has become reflective and less verbal in the relationship. Consequently, the stutterer no longer receives feedback and is unable to determine if the therapist understands and accepts this new behavior. The sessions devoted to superficial conversation then, are necessary to reassure the client that the therapist is still "with him."

Another change in the nature of the therapeutic interaction becomes apparent as the third stage progresses. Previous to the Introspection and Testing Stage, very little time was spent in discussing the stutterer's inter-personal relationships outside of the therapy situation. Now, however, the stutterer begins to discuss his relationships with his friends and colleagues and to illustrate his introspections with specific examples of his mode of interaction with others.

During the Introspection and Testing Stage, the therapist is called upon to discriminate between intellectualization and meaningful introspection on the part of the client. This has proven to be a difficult discrimination to make. In an attempt to control intellectualization, the therapist must continually press the stutterer for concrete examples of the feelings and dynamics the stutterer is discussing. If the stutterer is unable to relate a concept he is discussing to a meaningful concrete situation within his own experience, it may be assumed that he is intellectualizing. It is the therapist's task during the Introspection and Testing Stage to reward meaningful introspection on the part of the client and to prohibit intellectualization.

Another problem the therapist faces during this third stage in therapy is that of reacting to the stutterer's sudden expressions of ego strength. Typically, as the stutterer begins to understand himself and perceive others more accurately, he wishes to "correct" the situations he now perceives as being unrealistic. For example, one of the stutterers in therapy suddenly came to the realization that his employer was "using him." Before entering therapy, the stutterer had felt that the employer was being kind just to "put up with him." The stutterer's new perception of the situation appeared accurate to the therapist: the employer *was* "using" the client. In one therapy session, the stutterer informed his therapist that he had decided to "tell his boss off." Although the therapist was careful not to negate the feelings of the stutterer, the therapist, in discussing this case, noted that it was difficult not to restrain the client. In this case, the stutterer did tell his boss "off" and, as could be predicted, did receive better working conditions. Of course, not all expressions of new ego strength on the part of the stutterer will result in such good fortune as observed in the case noted above. It is important, however, that the therapist understands these expressions of growth and that he does not restrain the growth, unless, of course, the stutterer indicates some bizarre plan of action. In that case, it is doubtful if the plan of action of the part of the client is a result of growth toward self-actualization.

Therapists frequently observe that the client begins to indicate a new awareness of the therapist as the Introspection and Testing Stage continues. Clients, for example, may suddenly indicate a sincere desire to know about the therapist and his family. This is apparently related to the stutterer's heightened perceptions of himself and others. To be trite: now that the stutterer can look at himself, he can also observe others. Typically, the stutterer will report that the frequency and severity of his stuttering has diminished during this stage of therapy. This gradual lessening of stuttering is apparently related to the stutterer's more accurate perception of himself and of his relationships with others. It will be recalled that the Introspection and Testing Stage began with the client expressing negative affect toward the therapist. As this stage continues, with the stutterer engaged in introspection and in testing his new awareness of himself in situations outside of the therapeutic situation, the client's affect toward the therapist becomes more positive. Typically, the therapist's affect toward the client also becomes more positive. The Introspection and Testing Stage begins to terminate when the stutterer (now more capable of understanding himself and more capable of accurately perceiving himself and others) indicates that he is willing to assume the responsibility for determining what he must *do* to gain more satisfying relationships.

IV. Symptom Modification Stage

The Symptom Modification Stage commences when the stutterer, through his own decisions, seizes upon the structuring that the therapist did in the first stage of therapy and begins to modify that behavior which now seems inappropriate to the stutterer. This behavior on the part of the stutterer can only be explained in terms of the assumption that stutterers, like others, strive for self-actualization and have the capacity and the motivation to achieve wholeness.

It has already been noted that the frequency and severity of the stuttering has gradually diminished during the Introspection and Testing Stage of therapy. Frequently, however, mannerisms associated with the moment of stuttering continue through sheer habit strength. The stutterer now directs his attention to these and is capable of quickly overcoming those mannerisms which the stutterer feels continue to interfere with communication. It can also be observed that the stutterer begins to withdraw his emotional dependence on the therapist. As the stutterer strives for wholeness, he seeks *reciprocal* relationships outside of the therapeutic situation. The stutterer may announce in dramatic fashion that he no longer "needs" the therapist. Assuming that this statement is based on self-understanding and self-awareness, it is perhaps the best indication that therapy may be terminated. Another indicator of the terminal stage of therapy is that the stutterer notes that his attention has shifted from the nature of his speech in an inter-personal situation to the nature of the content of the inter-personal interaction. During this terminal stage of therapy, the client's affective attitudes toward the therapist become relatively stable and are generally more positive than at any previous time in therapy. As the stutterer begins to anticipate withdrawal from therapy, he may express a desire to discuss the therapeutic relationship. It is apparent that the client wishes to make closure on the relationship and needs to verbalize his feelings and reactions to what has taken place in the therapeutic situation.

Limitations

Inter-Personal Communications Therapy is admittedly in the developmental stage. To date, only a handful of clients have received therapy by therapists (other than the author) familiar with the rationale and procedures as outlined in this chapter. However, experienced therapists, when introduced to the IPC Therapy System of therapy, have frequently noted that, upon reflection, they can see how cases they have had "fit the pattern" of IPC Therapy. They report that, when therapy is presented in this fashion, they can see *post hoc* the progression of events which precipitated behavioral change in earlier cases. A research project is now underway to further delineate behavior in IPC Therapy and to evaluate in as objective a fashion as possible, the therapeutic successes and failures when IPC Therapy is employed.

Presently, IPC Therapy is presented as a system of therapy for use with stutterers. Because most authorities in speech pathology have acknowledged the importance of the therapeutic relationship with all types of speech disorders, it is conceivable that a system of therapy which is based on the manipulation of the therapeutic relationship will be constructed for each of the speech disorders. IPC Therapy, as presented here, is limited to use within an individual therapy situation. Research with groups under going a modified version of IPC Therapy is anticipated.

Because of the nature of the interaction between client and therapist, the frequency of therapy sessions plays a significant role in the speed with which a meaningful therapeutic interaction begins to take place. It is most advantageous to the development of a meaningful therapeutic relationship if therapy is scheduled as frequently as possible. Success has been achieved, however, with the frequency being limited to two one hour sessions weekly.

With how many stutterers does IPC Therapy appear appropriate? The developmental nature of IPC Therapy has been noted and no attempt will be made at present to explicitly state the qualifications of stutterers who could or could not benefit from the IPC system of therapy. To date, IPC Therapy has been used with adult (16 years and older) stutterers. It is assumed, although no research has been conducted to substantiate the observation, that IPC Therapy is most successful with stutterers with at least average intelligence.

IPC Therapy appears more relevant to those stutterers who perceive their stuttering as something (as Williams (15) has described it) that just happens and is, in a sense, perceived as an entity, an animistic "it" that does something to the stutterer. Through IPC Therapy, those stutterers who perceive their problem in terms of an "it" are forced into an emotional inter-personal involvement in which they evaluate this perception, and are guided to evaluate their stuttering as "inseparable to their being." An evaluation of the literature regarding stuttering indicates that a large percentage of the stutterers do enter therapy with the above noted perception.

Because IPC Therapy is based on the manipulation of the inter-personal interaction in the therapy situation, it does not appear an appropriate system to be used with those few stutterers who experience severe emotional disorders. Because the stutterer will perceive "threat" at various stages in the therapy, it is important that the stutterer has sufficient ego strength and emotional integrity (both terms admittedly vague but nevertheless meaningful to trained personnel) to undergo the treatment. Those few stutterers who possess only a tenuous grasp on purposeful behavior or are psychotic should, of course, be referred to a psychologist or a psychiatrist.

In IPC Therapy, the Diagnostic and Structuring Stage provides an opportunity for the therapist to assess the stutterers ego strength and emotional integrity before any threat (in IPC Therapy-Confrontation of behavior) is introduced in the relationship. It is difficult to state in explicit terms the dimensions of a stutterer's personality which would indicate that the stutterer cannot accept and benefit from IPC Therapy. Through observation of the stutterer in the Diagnostic and Structuring Stage, however, the therapist becomes aware of any bizarre behavior and attitudes indicative of a severe emotional disorder. If the therapist experiences difficulty in communicating to the stutterer the rather concrete concepts utilized in IPC Therapy in the Diagnostic and Structuring Stage, the ability of the stutterer to benefit from IPC Therapy may be seriously questioned. For example, stutterers with severe emotional disorders are frequently involved in themselves to such an extent that the therapist cannot communicate the structuring of therapy to them.

Implications

The success of a therapy system based on the manipulation of the therapeutic relationship is dependent to a large extent upon the therapist's ability to function adequately in varying types of interpersonal relationships. This skill, obviously, is difficult to learn, and has led many to discuss at length whether a good therapist is "born" or "trained" or both. After reviewing the literature relative to the qualities associated with a good therapist, it was concluded that Barbara's (2) discussion regarding the essential competencies of a "stuttering therapist" was not only pertinent, but appropriate to the needs of IPC Therapy. Briefly stated, Barbara holds that a therapist should:

a. Have his own personal problems reasonably well resolved, or be sufficiently aware of them so as to control their effect in the relationship.
b. Be integrated enough to handle most eventualities in the therapeutic relationship and (of particular relevance to IPC Therapy) be able to handle his own reaction anxieties and hostilities without harming the patient.
c. Hold an inherent belief in man's ability to grow toward self-actualization.
d. Be trained and well oriented in the dynamics of human behavior.
e. Have an awareness of and an understanding for the person who stutters.
f. Be, in every aspect of his personality, a human being — capable of feeling for struggle and suffering in humans.

Because of the nature of IPC Therapy, the question will arise as to whether it should be conducted by a speech pathologist or a psychologist. There is no simple answer for this question. Training of speech pathologists today generally includes an extensive background both in the theory and practice of psychotherapy. Conversely, the training of psychologists generally includes at least a perfunctory introduction to the analysis of abnormal speech symptomalogy. In practice, therapy for adult stutterers generally is conducted by persons either in speech pathology or psychology who have indicated a particular interest and skill in handling the problem. The assumption is made that IPC Therapy can be conducted by speech therapists possessing qualities similar to those noted by Barbara (2) and reviewed above, and by Psychologists who are capable of identifying and understanding the overt stuttering symptomatology.

IPC Therapy was constructed in such a fashion as to be consistent with principles of learning. To be consistent with learning principles, a system must suggest that the client's behavior be manipulated and controlled. Skinner (12) and Frank (7) noted that people influence and control one another in any inter-personal interaction. IPC Therapy attempts to control and manipulate the client in a systematic fashion to facilitate client growth. Bandura (1) reviewed current forms of therapy in terms of the learning process and concluded that many of the changes observed in psychotherapy can be accounted for in terms of the therapist's direct reward and punishment of the client's expressions. IPC Therapy is based on the assumption that the therapist rewards and punishes varying client responses depending upon the stage of therapy attained. For example, during the *Examination and Confrontation Stage,* the consistently "punishes" such behavior as intellectualization, denial, and avoidance, and consistently rewards such behavior as introspection, verbalization of feeling, and affective display. In total, the therapist's behavior creates a learning experience for the stutterer in an inter-personal relationship. Bendura (1) noted that the role assumed by therapists using currently popular forms of psychotherapy may bring the therapist many direct or fantasied personal gratifications. On the other hand, Bandura observed that therapy derived from learning theory places the therapist in a less glamorous role. He noted that this may create some reluctance on the part of therapists to part with the more glamorous procedures currently in use.

Summary

A system of stuttering therapy utilizing the concept of inter-personal communications as the basic factor has been proposed. Inter-Personal Communications Therapy (IPC Therapy) is based on the concept that through the control and manipulation of the therapeutic relationship, the stutterer undergoes a meaningful learning experience in inter-personal relationships which enables the stutterer to modify that behavior which was reinforced and maintained through distorted perceptions of inter-personal relationships. IPC Therapy was presented as a process having four stages: *I. Diagnostic and Structuring, II. Examination and Confrontation, III. Introspection and Testing,* and *IV. Symptom Modification.* Following the presentation of these four stages, a discussion of IPC Therapy's limitations and implications was presented.

Bibliography

1. Bandura, A.: Psychotherapy as a learning process. *Psychological Bulletin, 58*:143-157, 1961.
2. Barbara, D.: *Stuttering: A Psychodynamic Approach to its Understanding and Treatment.* New York, Julian Press, 1954.
3. Bloodstein, O.: Stuttering as an anticipatory struggle reaction, in *Stuttering: A Symposium.* New York, Harper and Brothers, 1958.
4. Combs, A. W. and Snygg, D.: *Individual Behavior. A Perceptual Approach to Behavior.* New York, Harper and Brothers, 1959.
5. Cooper, E. B.: *Patient therapist relationships and concomitent factors in stuttering therapy.* Doctoral Thesis, The Pennsylvania State University, 1962.
6. Diehl, C. F.: Patient-therapist relationship, in *The Psychotherapy of Stuttering.* Springfield, Thomas, 1962.
7. Frank, J. D.: The dynamics of the psychotherapeutic relationship, *Psychiatry, 22*:17-39, 1959.
8. Martin, E. W.: Client centered therapy as a theoretical orientation for speech therapy. *Asha, 5*:576-578, 1963.
9. Murphy, A. T. and FitzSimons, R. M.: *Stuttering andd Personality Dynamics.* New York, The Ronald Press, 1960.
10. Rogers, C. R.: *Client-Centered Therapy.* New York, Houghton Mifflin, 1951.

11. Sheehan, J. G.: Conflict theory of stuttering, in *Stuttering: A Symposium.* New York, Harper and Brothers, 1958.

12. Skinner, B. F.: Some issues concerning the control of human behavior. *Science, 124*:1057-1066, 1956.

13. Snyder, W. and Snyder, J.: *The Psychotherapy Relationship.* New York, Macmillan Company, 1961.

14. Van Riper, C.: *Speech Correction, Prinicples and Methods.* Englewood Cliffs, N. J., Prentice-Hall Inc., 1963.

15. Williams, D. E.: A point of view about stuttering. *Speech Hearing Dis., 22*:390-397 1957.

6

The Self as a Central Concept in Speech Therapy for the Person Who Stutters

Edwin W. Martin, Ph.D.
Louise M. Ward, M.A.
T. Earle Johnson, Ph.D.

Speech therapists have been implored, repeatedly, to treat the whole person. So much so, in fact, that it seems to be generally agreed that the whole person is being treated. Yet the mechanics for treatment of the whole person through speech therapy are for the most part unspecified. How, in fact, might "the whole person" be treated?

One possibility is to departmentalize the treatment process. The speech therapist can work with the speech, in the present case, stuttering. Other problems dealing with interpersonal relationships and the use of speech can be referred to the psychiatrist and the psychologist.

In everyday experience this solution seems lacking. The nature of speech behavior seems to link it closely with the total responses of the organism. This is seen particularly clearly in relation to stuttering where the effects of changes in the meaning of situations for the individual are reflected in variations in his speech behavior. Recognition of this relationship between whole and sub-part has been reflected in various treatment procedures ranging in emphasis from psychoanalysis to direct symptom modification. Van Riper (20) has written of the gains in personality adjustment possible through symptomatic treatment of stuttering. Johnson (11) and Williams (22), while rejecting a "neurotic" theory of causation of stuttering have concerned themselves with the perceptual and evaluative response of the speaker. Sheehan (16) suggests an integration of speech therapy and psychotherapy through a "conflict theory" of stuttering. Virtually every reference to therapy for stuttering in the literature attempts to come to terms with this issue, either through definition of the problem or treatment methods.

If we eliminate from our thinking for the moment positions which might be conceived as polar, i.e., non-symptomatic approaches, and strictly symptom-oriented approaches, we are left with a broad middle ground. In this middle ground seems to fall the bulk of the literature on the treatment of stuttering. Here we find the accumulation of experience and theorizing of numbers of scholar-clinicians, and a multitude of divergent techniques.

We are faced, then, with this situation. We are interested in treating the person who stutters in the most effective manner possible. For most authors this implies a recognition of the whole individual and interactions with sub-parts, speech behavior and stuttering. It is recognized that certain individuals may have problems calling for referral to other sources of psychotherapeutic aid, but clinical experience and the bulk of experimental findings suggest that these are exceptions rather than the rule. Therefore, it seems imperative that we have a theory of therapy, or at least a conceptual framework, within which we can deal with the person who stutters, where he now is, including modification of his speech behavior and other relevant aspects of his behavior, such as feelings, attitudes, perceptions, etc. Such a conceptual framework should be related to the mass of current knowledge on treatment of stuttering and also provide a direction for increasing understanding of the therapeutic relationship.

The concept of "self" which has played an important part in various theories of personality, and which has been mentioned in a variety of contexts in the speech pathology literature on stuttering, seems to offer a possibility for such a conceptual framework. Hall and Lindzey (9) have commented:

The term *self* as used in modern psychology has come to have two distinct meanings. On the one hand it is defined as the person's attitudes and feelings about himself, and on the other hand it is regarded as a group of psychological processes which govern behavior and adjustment . . . It should be pointed out and clearly understood that no modern theory of the self holds that there is a psychic agent or "inner manikin" which regulates man's action . . . In other words, the self is not a metaphysical or religious concept; it is a concept that falls within the domain of a scientific psychology (p. 468).

The concept of self as used in this paper has roots in the "Field Theory" of Kurt Lewin (12) and the related "Interpersonal" theory of Sullivan (18) among others, and has been synthesized in the writing of Carl Rogers (15). In Rogers' theoretical schema there are three principal ingredients: a) the organism, or individual; b) the phenomenal field, or total experience of the individual, and c) the self, or the part of the "field" consisting of a conceptual pattern of perceptions of characteristics and relationships of the "I" or the "me," together with the values attached to these concepts.

"The organism," says Rogers, "has one basic tendency and striving—to actualize, maintain, and enhance the experiencing organism" (p. 487). This is seen as a directional movement toward what might be called maturity and greater independence. Also Rogers said, "the self-actualization of the organism appears to be in the direction of socialization, broadly defined" (p. 488). This basic concept, that man strives in the direction of a positive or growth dimension, occurs in the writings of a number of personality theorists, Sullivan (18), Horney (10), Goldstein (8), Snygg and Combs (17), etc.

If we look at the role of the self in relation to the phenomenal field and the organism, we see that the self is not synonymous with the organism, it represents an abstraction of the phenomenal field organism. It is those parts of the organism and its experiences which are conceived as the "I" or "me," the awareness of being, of functioning. The conception of the self and of the self in relation to others also includes a value system giving positive or negative weight to its qualities and experiences. The positive and negative values may arise directly out of the experience of the individual and also may be by introjection taken over from others.

The significance of the self may be seen in Rogers' statement, "Most of the ways of behaving which are adopted by the organism are those which are consistent with the concept of self" (p. 507). If we are interested in changing behavior, then, we become involved in the relationship of the behavior to the self-concept of the individual. For example, does the new desired behavior, i.e., fluency, fit the conception of self?

Rogers commented additionally that some behavior may be brought about by organic experiences and needs which are not in the conscious awareness of the individual, "but in such instances the behavior is not 'owned' by the individual" (p. 509). Here again the relationship to therapy for stuttering may be seen. Williams (22) has approached this subject in his discussion of the "it" connected with stuttering. He pointed out the frequent personification of stuttering, and encouraged the person who stutters to see the stuttering as behavior which the stutterer is engaged in and not as something which is happening to him.

As an individual experiences events in life he may respond by giving these experiences meaning, i.e., symbolizing them and then organizing them into some relationship to the self; he may ignore them because they are not perceived as pertinent to the self; or he may deny them symbolization or give them distorted symbolization because the experiences are inconsistent with the structure of the self.

In summary, we see the self as a differentiated part of the experiencing organism, those parts conceived as the "I" or "me." In a sense, the self may act as a criterion against which the organism places its experiences. Those which "fit" are symbolized and included, others are essentially ignored, still others are denied or distorted. To the extent the organism must deny or distort significant experiences it is "mal-adjusted."

The literature on speech pathology contains numerous references to the self in a variety of contexts, and with a variety of meanings. In discussing therapeutic procedures, authors with theories of etiology as diverse as West, Eisenson, Glauber and Bloodstein, for example, include references to the self.

Bloodstein (4), in discussing learning to speak about stuttering "freely and frankly" to others, remarked, "Self-acceptance . . . is a most vital part of any type of personal adjustment" (p. 45). Glauber (7) commented, ". . . speech is the self in action; the self exposed in the acting out of an instinctual drive" (p. 79). In discussing the "self-images of the stutterer" he added, "the feeling about the self . . . are those of incompleteness, separatedness, helplessness, even of self-destruction" (p. 105).

West (21) suggested, "the stutterer's attitude toward himself must be changed" (p. 211). Eisenson (6) emphasized self-acceptance as a part of therapy for the "organic stutterer." He discussed the need for therapy activities promoting objective evaluation and acceptance of perseverative language usage, and said, "through this approach (the therapist) helps the stutterer to self-acceptance . . ." Shearer (15a), Murphy and Fitzsimons (14a), and Clark and Fitzpatrick (4a) have presented extensive discussions of the self as a construct in diagnosis and treatment of stuttering.

The present chapter attributes to the self the central role in mediating the individual's behavior and presents a viewpoint that experiences of the self are a basic therapeutic process.

Therapy for Adults Who Stutter

A therapy program for adults, using the self as a central concept, might be seen as having two broad aspects, each designed to promote enhancement of the self. These aspects are not dichotomized in actual practice, rather they seem to overlap and interact. The first aspect is centered around speech production, per se, and deals with observation of and experimentation with speech behavior and associated thoughts and feelings. The second aspect consists of activities designed specifically to strengthen the ability of the individual to assimilate into his self more of his experiences. This latter aspect may be more clearly understood in relation to the conception, discussed earlier, that "mal-adjustment" may be defined in terms of the extent an individual needs to deny his experiences awareness because they are incongruent with his self-concept.

Speech Production Activities

The emphasis in speech production activities is on observation and experimentation. Observing and experimenting are seen as continuing processes and the therapist attempts to help the client develop an "attitude" of observation and experimentation. The individual is felt to have the capacity for observing and modifying speech behavior, but generally has had reduced ability to perceive and assimilate his experiences in these areas.

OBSERVATION

Beginning work on observation may be pointed toward the parts of the speech act which may be seen or heard by others, i.e., repetition of sounds, prolongations, tongue protrusion, etc. Attention can also be given to what the client feels is going on within himself on a physical basis, i.e., tension in stomach, tongue against alveolar ridge, etc. During this process the therapist and the client can discuss these observations in terms of "what the client *is doing*," not what is happening "*to him.*" This emphasis on what might be called acceptance of the responsibility for behaving in the manner called "stuttering" has its roots in Williams' "Point of View About Stuttering" (22).

The question may be raised, "What is therapeutic about the activities of observing?" Value may be found in the facilitation of observation as the individual becomes more able to perceive his behavior and to handle his perceptions consciously. Further, the relationship between the client and the therapist as they discuss the observations has therapeutic potentiality.

The therapist has the opportunity while discussing the client's observations of his speech behavior to understand as nearly as possible, the client's "world" (phenomenal field). With this understanding he attempts to communicate an acceptance for the client. This emphasis on understanding and acceptance as the basis of psychotherapy has been presented by Rogers (15). Martin (13) pointed out that understanding and acceptance are not necessarily limited to material presented in counseling, but rather can be used by speech therapists countless times during the therapeutic relationship. As the person who stutters attempts to observe his behavior the therapist can communicate much understanding and acceptance in the attempt to share with the client what he is doing while he is stuttering.

A need for therapists to "understand" what it is like to stutter has been pointed out in the literature. There have been suggestions that student-clinicians psuedo-stutter in public situations and attain more "feeling for" the person who stutters. Others have suggested the therapist and client witness the therapist stuttering in stores, etc. and observe the reaction of the other persons involved. These activities seem to have been planned to enlarge the understanding of either therapist or client as to the reactions of the person who stutters and of the listener. What has been suggested in the preceding discussion is that such activities may well serve this purpose and also serve the purpose of the basic understanding relationship between therapist and client.

Martin (13) discussed an example of Van Riper making an initial contact with a boy who stuttered. Van Riper sat close to the boy and elicited from him what he did when he stuttered and then attempted to feel the same tensions in his speaking mechanisms. As he did he checked with the boy to see if he was reproducing the stuttering accurately. His voice was calm and he communicated an interest in understanding. Afterwards, observers were struck by the liason between the two.

Activities designed to facilitate observation do not need to be focused only on negative aspects of the speaking process. We can also observe things which the speaker can do, and perhaps, more important, likes. Many persons with speech problems, not just people who stutter, tend to regard their speech as exaggeratedly poor. We have asked numbers of our clients to rate their speech on such variables as accuracy of articulation, intelligibility, pleasantness, ability to communicate, etc. They use a regular percentage scale 0 to 100 per cent and generally conform to an academic grading system 70-75 being fair, 90-100 excellent, etc. Few grade themselves higher than 70-75 on any aspect of their speech, even when other judges grade some aspects, for example, articulation, as "good" or "excellent." Many grade themselves as poor in all aspects without differentiation. This negative "halo effect" can frequently be reduced as an individual becomes more aware of the several aspects of his speaking and more accurately pinpoints his difficulties. In group work other clients are particularly quick to notice good aspects of another's speech.

Along with attention to the speaking process the therapist can focus attention on what might be called the communication dimension, i.e., "Is the message of the speaker being understood?" Numerous clients have verbalized doubt that they are understood; that they can get their message across. Perhaps a classic example was a college professor who had been teaching ten years, yet had basic doubts about the ability of his speech to be understood.

In summary, activities designed to help the client observe his speech may have all the traditional values placed on them, i.e., developing more accurate perceptions, gaining a more "objective" point of view, etc. These activities also provide an excellent opportunity for the therapist to respond to the client with an attitude of understanding and acceptance. Basic to this attitude must be the assumption on the part of the therapist that the client will have a tendency to move toward growth naturally, and that the therapist may further this progress through an approach which emphasizes understanding. It is not necessary for the therapist to "drive" the client toward growth.

Experimentation: Along with increased attention on what he is doing, the client is urged to experiment with his speaking, and then to discuss with the therapist his observations and evaluations concerning his experiments. In this process, as well as in observation, aspects of the conversational interchange which were judged to be positive, as well as negative, are discussed.

Including emphasis on positive behavior is not an attempt to "brainwash" the person into believing his speech is good; it is rather an attempt to help him develop a concept of himself that would include adequacy connected with speaking. As a person begins to feel he has some strengths as a speaker and as a person, he is often more able to view his weaknesses realistically. A young man who was showing very little progress in changing his speech was particularly resistant to using a tape recorder to observe his speech. It was felt that his concept of his speech and of himself as a speaker was so poor that such observation was too painful for him. The therapists worked with him on picking some aspects of his speech which he felt were satisfactory. He practiced saying several phrases paying particular attention to whether they were understandable, had pleasant vocal quality, etc. When he began to feel more positive about his efforts, he was willing to tape these phrases and then invited several staff members to listen to how well he was doing.

Williams (22) spoke of developing a concept of fluency. He urged that the speaker study fluency and develop an awareness of his own fluency so that he can "picture it," in a sense, and develop the ability to speak naturally, rather than "not stutter." His approach seems to parallel the activities reported above, which are not restricted to fluency, and we find it well suited to use as an activity for experimentation.

A primary emphasis in experimentation is on activities which strive to enhance the individual's concept of himself. What we are interested in first is the person. His speech should serve him. If an individual wants a cup of coffee, his speech should help him get it. If he winds up with milk because he could say milk, the individual suffers. His concept of himself is reduced and he is the slave to his speech.

Urging the individual who stutters to ask for the coffee, stuttering or not, has been recommended frequently by numerous therapists for a variety of theoretic reasons; it might be seen, for example, as strengthening an "approach" tendency by Sheehan (16). It has been our experience that when an individual asks for what he wants, or behaves in a similar fashion in other challenging situations, and when he feels some satisfaction from his efforts, he seems to have had an important therapeutic experience. In self-theory terminology, the individual has contacted the environment and has evaluated the outcome as consistent with a more positive conception of self.

In addition to choosing activities because they offer the possibility of strengthening positive self-regard, the therapist must ask himself what happens if the activity is not an immediate success. Suppose in asking for the coffee, the individual becomes so "blocked" that he stands mute for long seconds, finally squeezing out a partially intelligible grunt, which the clerk correctly interprets, before the client moves embarrassedly away. Is this activity therapeutic? Is the client told, "Well, if at first you don't succeed . . ."?

Here we can see clearly the interaction between the therapeutic relationship and the activities which are placed on this foundation. This is where the concept "experimentation" may have real meaning. If a therapeutic relationship has been established where the emphasis is on communication, understanding, acceptance of the individual, this experience does not have to be a disaster.

First, the goal for the activity need not be structured solely in terms of fluency, ease, etc. While it is hoped that the client will experience success in the activity, in terms of getting his needs met, the activity is seen as an experiment. It is, in a sense, grist for the mill; something to observe, something to try out, something to communicate about.

While it is unrealistic to assume that an individual can develop an "experimental immunity" or "objectivity" so that he is totally free from pain in failure, it does seem true that such pain may be reduced by appropriate goal setting. It must be emphasized here that the therapist must see this process of client and therapist planning activities to be experimented with and discussed as the essence of the therapy. If he believes in the technique, per se, the client will tend to do so also.

In contrast, it often seems as though the sharing of a painful experience can promote the progress of therapy. If through the therapeutic interaction surrounding such an event the client can maintain his feelings in awareness and integrate these feelings into his self-structure a surface-level failure can be a more basic success. In this situation the therapist has an opportunity to communicate understanding and acceptance which can cut through the client's feelings of isolation and despair and so help him "live through" the experience without needing to distort it perceptually or deny it to awareness.

The activities in which the client engages as he observes and experiments are selected for the most part by the client. Early in the relationship the therapist may suggest several alternatives the client may choose from, but the emphasis is on client initiative and choice. Activities may consist of words or phrases used in everyday speech, or situations such as telephoning, ordering in a restaurant, "small-talking," etc.

In summary, examples of speech behavior from the everyday conversation of the client are chosen to serve as objects for observation and experimentation. The observation may serve to help the client develop a more accurate perception of his speech and his feelings connected with his speech. The speech behavior moves from the unknowable toward the knowable. Similarly, in experimentation the client may try a range of behavior designed to help him develop a sense of power or control in communication situations. He may work toward developing a concept of fluency, or generalized speech adequacy. In each situation emphasis is placed on behaving in ways which he judges as worthy of self-respect and which can provide him with a sense of satisfaction. Underlying all these activities is his continuing relationship with the therapist. The therapist tries to make this relationship empathicly understanding, and to communicate this understanding and regard to the client.

Experience of the Self as a Whole

It may be seen that the aspects of therapy discussed above, while concerning themselves directly with modification of speech behavior, are also designed to provide for experiencing the self as a whole. Other activities, not focused directly on speech modification may be designed specifically to implement the experiencing of self.

Included in the program for adults are activities such as group role-playing and discussions, counseling, social hours, recreation, and also creative activities such as painting, modeling, etc. Use of such activities in group speech therapy has been discussed by Backus (2) as possessing potentiality for strengthening self-regard and increasing self-understanding.

Of particular interest has been the use of role-playing to facilitate self-understanding and to provide a medium for self-expression. As we have defined it role-playing has its origins in the psychodrama of Moreno (14). We have attempted to modify Moreno's procedures by putting the activities within a framework which we felt was consistent with "client-centered" therapy. For example, there is little emphasis on interpretation, less speaking for the client by "doubles," more reliance on the client to choose situations for playing, etc.

As clients play out situations which concern them, or in which they felt success there is no effort by therapists to modify or call attention to speech behavior. Responses are primarily attempts to understand feelings, questions to group members about their impressions, etc.

Frequently clients will choose activities to play where they will want to express themselves or assert themselves as individuals. Examples of such activities include: arguing with a parent about use of the family car, or dating; returning defective merchandise, asking for a date, applying for a job, etc. Another favorite activity is being "any one you want." A basic characteristic of the performances and subsequent discussions of these role-playing situations is the quest of the individual to feel a sense of power, a sense of "I can," as opposed to powerlessness. Although there are numerous comments about speech, reflecting on increases or decreases in fluency, much attention is given to the overall goal of the total individual, "I got what I wanted," or "I wanted to say what I felt, but I decided to play it safe."

Clients seem to use role-playing as an intermediary between clinic practice activities and "real life." The actual feelings stirred by the role-playing provide reality elements and yet there is also a dimension of "within-the-clinic-security." These activities may represent a less complex or simplified everyday life. Often after role-playing a client will report he repeated the activity in the outside world, asking for a date, confronting a stranger, etc. Almost always these experiences are felt to be successful.

Although role-playing as discussed above is conducted for the experience itself and its psychotherapeutic potential, modified role-playing can be the basis for speech production activities. Frequently a client will want to continue an activity for several days, while he concentrates on his speech behavior during the activity, his swings of feeling, etc.

Role-playing and the other activities mentioned, social hours, recreation, etc., are seen as therapy activities in which the inner potentialities of an individual are given a chance for expression. The strengths of an individual are believed to be potentially present and the drive for "growth" intrinsic; the role of therapy is to provide an opportunity for experimenting, observing and succeding.

Summary

A client reports, "I am talking in staff conferences. Occasionally I stutter, but the others are more interested in what I have to say than how I say it." He seems to have both a realistic and positive regard for himself and his speech usage. Another client in recalling a day at work he felt pleased about, reported that he had given good service, that he had felt satisfied that he had been understood and had communicated well. When he reported failures he talked in terms of fluency seemingly equating stuttering and himself; successes were seen in somewhat broader terms, professional competency and self-expression.

These examples are used to illustrate that stuttering must be seen in terms of its meaning for the individual, how he relates it to himself. Activities designed to promote speech change and related change in feelings, attitudes, etc., can use the self as a central concept, as a representation of the basic organism, "the whole person." Fundamental to positive change in the individual is an increased ability to perceive accurately, and to assimilate experiences into the self. Speech therapy should be designed to provide an opportunity for observation and experimentation within a climate of understanding and acceptance.

Therapy as Experiences of Self for Children Who Stutter

A child is born into a system of relationships. These relationships include relationship with one's self, with others and with the total environment. In and through this system of relationships he must come to experience himself as a self. It is the dynamic self-affirmation of life that a being strives to experience himself with ever increasing intensiveness and extensiveness. Thus a child grows. It is in a balance of appropriate intensiveness and extensiveness of his experience of himself that normal development lies. Through increasing intensiveness his experience of self gains depth while through extensiveness it gains scope. He must experience himself intensively as an individual and also experience himself extensively as a part, a part of a group and a part of his total environment. He must experience intensively the parts of himself, the various functions of himself. He must also experience extensively himself as a whole, as undissected, undetermined, a unity while yet a diversity.

His experience of himself is extended to include verbal behavior as one vehicle of his self-affirmation. When a child stutterers some break has occurred in the normal progression of his experience of himself. Wherever this occurred originally it comes to affect the way he experiences himself as a self as well as in relation to others and to the total environment. Therapy, then, becomes a system of experiences of self which can re-establish the normal progression of actualizing himself with increasing intensiveness and extensiveness.

An attempt will be made here to describe therapy for children as such a system of experiences of self.

This section has three parts: Clinical Format, The Intensive Experience of Being One's Self, and The Extensive Experience of Being a Part.

Clinical Format

This particular format has been developed in a University training clinic where advanced student therapists work with a clinical supervisor. Children have attended two hour daily sessions during a five or six week block of time. Children usually attend two or three six week blocks during a year. In some cases, once a week therapy periods have continued in the interim months between the six week blocks; however, most children are seen only in the concentrated session. Consultation with and/or referral to the University psychological clinic has been available.

There are three important characteristics of this format which may be adapted for use in other clinics and public schools where one therapist is working alone. The first characteristic is the combination of group and individual experience in therapy providing for the bi-polar nature of experience as an individual and experience as a participant. The importance of an appropriate balance in this two-fold relationship has been stressed by many thinkers concerned with the human situation. Thus, a child in his particularity and in his individual character seems one important focus in the system of experiences that make up therapy. The successful experience of self as a part of a group also needs the guidance and special provision for healing experience which therapy can provide. In clinical settings where one therapist works alone this has been handled by seeing children individually before and after the group periods.

The second characteristic considered to be important is the combination of activities focused on the particularities of the speech

symptoms and activities focused on providing more holistic communicative experiences, such as play therapy, role playing, refresh-
ment time, etc. This division concerns the content dimension of
therapy situations as opposed to their personal and interpersonal
structure.

The third characteristic is the concentration in time of the therapy experience. Choosing to concentrate therapy into daily intensive
experiences for discrete blocks of time rather than to diffuse it
over longer periods of time seems to have advantages for effecting
changes in behavior. It provides a barrage of experience with a
positive dynamic force which has been found to have a lasting
effect.

The Intensive Experience of Being One's Self

During two periods which make up about half of each clinic
day, a child is alone in a small room with his individual therapist.
Here the focus is on the child as a separate, individual, self-determining self. Although he obviously experiences himself in relation
to the therapist, he or she is there to serve the child, to facilitate his
individual experiencing of himself. During these two periods, two
types of situations are provided. One is designed to facilitate the
extensive experience of himself as a whole; that is, a more complete, more integrated, more self-affirming experience of himself
as a whole. The other is designed to facilitate the intensive experience as a part of himself; that is, to facilitate his experiencing of
the specific part functioning speech. A play therapy type situation
provides for the extensive experience of himself as a whole. The
speech-centered situation provides for the intensive experience of
a part of himself. But both concern individualization as opposed to
participation.

A client-centered approach to play therapy has been taken. Detailed discussion of this approach has been published by Axline
(1), and Dorfman (5). The therapist attempts to maintain: a)
a high degree of congruence in his own being; b) an unconditioned
positive regard for the child, and c) a deep, empathic understanding
of the child. This situation is considered to provide the child a
highly simplified relationship and a highly simplified communicative situation. The child as a whole is met with attitudes of accep-

tance, deep respect for his intrinsic worth and faith in his self-determining potential. He is free to choose his own activity within the limits of the playroom. He is free to speak or not to speak. His expressions are given a positive feed-back of the most adequate and simplified reflection by the therapist. Limitations on his total expression of whatever he is are kept to that minimum which roots the experience in reality. Such an experience, which is focused on the child's free, open, spontaneous expression of his whole being, tends to expand his experiencing of himself to include more of his total experience and to integrate this experience into a unified self system.

Another dimension of the intensive experience of being one's self is the speech-centered situation. This dimension provides an intensive experience of a part of himself. The part function of speech is the focus. The kind and amount of focus given to the child's speech moves along a range with the age of the child as well as the severity and duration in time of the stuttering behavior. Speech activities used for the range of kind and amount of focus on speech behavior fall roughly into three categories. Categories by definition are based on similarities and bear the limitation that the differences of any individual child may break the applicability of the category. If it is kept in mind that their function is to bring order to a realm of experience perhaps these three may be useful to this discussion.

The first category of speech activity applies mostly to preschool children. The questions involved in taking for therapy preschool children who stutter have seemed to the writers to reside more in what kind of therapy is provided than in whether therapy is indicated. In this case the therapist engages with the child in some kind of activity which the child enjoys and which is apt to elicit verbal behavior. The therapist acts as a speech model providing positive feed-back for the child's speech in a very simplified form. This type of verbal situation has been described by Gertrud Wyatt (23). If the child's language is simple, the therapist's verbalizations may be slightly, but only slightly, more complex. If his language is highly complex, the therapist's language may be much simpler than his in order to bring him back to a level of language usage which he can handle successfully. The emphasis is on providing the best conditions for speech and language usage and not on the stuttering behavior.

The second category of speech activity is used when the stuttering pattern has progressed in consistency and severity to a point where the child has symbolized it as a speech difficulty, or he would have were he not denying it to his awareness. Activities in this category have two goals: a) to provide for the experience of fluency, and b) to prevent disowning of the stuttering behavior as a part of the self. These activities are built around conversational situations usually involving toys chosen for their appropriateness for repeated use of the same conversational speech responses; for example, in playing "store" such responses as, "May I help you?" "Yes, I'd like to buy some———." "That will be 20¢," etc. The repeated patterns mean that the child is engaging in an interactive communicative situation in which he can experience fluency. His experience of fluency is faciliated by the therapy. If the child does not observe stuttering when it occurs, the therapist may occasionally mention it, simply and with acceptance. The child is not pushed to observe the stuttering behavior, but often if the therapist simply states that this has occurred, he also begins to mention it.

The third category of speech activity applies mostly to children in middle and later elementary grades. It has similarities to the second, but progresses beyond it. It retains and builds upon the goals of the second, that is, providing an experience of fluency and preventing disowning of the stuttering. It goes on to the third goal of preventing of disowning of fluency and a fourth of helping the child to deal with the stuttering. It uses a conversational situation appropriate to this age child. These may be similar to the example in category two, but often deal with particular difficulties in speech situations, such as talking to school principals, giving messages, buying items in a store. Wherever possible these are extended out into real situations, such as actually delivering a message or actually going on a buying expedition. In these activities emphasis is placed on observation and experimentation with the stuttering behavior, with ways of "taking it easy," while also helping the child to be aware of times that he experiences fluency.

The fluid quality of these categories becomes apparent, that is, with any given child one may move backward or forward in this progression to meet the child where he is. In any case, the speech centered activities are chosen to provide experience with the part function of speech which are appropriate to the child's functioning as a totality.

To summarize, then, the child's intensive experience of being himself is conceived in two equally important and mutually dependent dimensions—the extensive experience of self as a whole and the intensive experience of a part of himself.

The Extensive Experience of Being a Part

Group experience in a program of therapy represents the other pole of the bi-polar nature of man's self-affirmation. Paul Tillich (19) has said,

> Man's self-affirmation has two sides which are distinguishable but not separable. One is the affirmation of the self as a self; that it, of a separate, self-centered, individualized, incomparable, free, self-determining self. That is what one affirms in every act of self-affirmation . . . But the self is self only because it has a world, a structured universe, to which it belongs and from which it is separated at the same time. Self and World are correlated and so are individualization and participation.

While the use of speech is rooted in being a differentiated self, and does not appear until a child has accomplished a certain degree of differentiation of the self, it also mediates his experience as a part of a group. Experience in therapy, then, should provide for this transition. The child moves from the individual situation into a group of four and five other children accompanied by his individual therapist, who remains in the group. The two daily group activities express the two dimensions of focus on the total functioning organism: a) the extensive experience of self as a whole, which is also a participant, and b) the intensive experience of part of the self, which is also participating.

The activity which has been most commonly used to provide experience of self as a whole, while participating in a group, is role-playing. As with adults, role-playing provides opportunity for children to give form to their thoughts, feelings and experiences, both verbally and nonverbally. This activity is structured by the therapist, although the children play a major role in the selection of situations and roles to be played. The three steps one finds outlined in the literature on role-playing are warm-up, acting out, and discussion. These have been followed with modification; for example, with young children and some older groups with speech difficulties it often seems wise to minimize or dispense with the discussions after acting out.

With young children, four, five and six years old, familiar fairy tales may serve as the situation with the children choosing different roles and often modifing the story to suit their choice of roles. For example, one group used the Cindrella story over and over again with their creation from this base bearing little resemblance to the original story. Judging from their interest and increased expressiveness, they were finding this story a meaningful skeleton around which they could express whatever they chose. Family situations and authority relationships such as those involving policemen, teachers, kings and queens, are often chosen for acting out. It is not unusual for older children to choose play situations involving their speech difficulty, such as being laughed at or not being understood.

The children's use of speech and absence of speech in role-playing is quite revealing. Children will often create nonverbal roles for themselves as their first attempts to participate. For example, one child suggested the inclusion of a puppy in a family situation and was willing to play this role before he was willing to play that of a family member. Marked differences in the stuttering behavior are often observed as children play different roles. For example, one boy stuttered more severely in playing an authority role, such as a policeman, than in any other situation in which he was observed. He seemed to delight in such roles, however, and chose such a role at every opportunity. After a few weeks, severe stuttering in authority roles subsided, and along with this change, he was noted to choose authority roles less often.

The therapist's response to the ways children choose and express their roles is non-evaluative, that is, he does not judge their performance as "good or bad," right or wrong. This non-evaluative response and the variety of possibilities open for different types and complexity of communication offers opportunity for children who participate to experience relative success.

The group activities in which speech is the focus follow the progression of roles described for the individual speech activities; that is: a) providing a verbal situation in which the level of speech and language usage is simple enough that the child can handle it; b) providing for the experience of fluency while attempting to prevent the child from disowning the stuttering, and c) preventing the disowning of fluency while helping him to deal more effectively with the stuttering. In the group situation as in the individual, the goals build on each other and progress with the age of the child and the severity of the stuttering. As in the experience of other workers, few of the children who begin treatment at preschool age are still in need of therapy in the school years if treatment has been followed through.

The use of speech is structured around a group activity appropriate to the age of the child and in which children would normally take turns and use conversational speech patterns. Backus and Beasley (3) have described similar group speech activities.

The interaction with the other children who are not there just to serve one child's needs as with the therapist in the individual speech situation, make this a more complex dynamic speech situation, yet it is kept simple for the child in that: a) activities come to have a familiar over-all pattern; b) his turn at speaking and serving as group leader is protected, and c) the repetition of a particular conversation pattern gives him a sureness of what is appropriate to say. Thus, he has certain securities within the dynamics and risks of group interaction.

Experience with children demonstrates that, properly guided, they facilitate each other's experiences of self in ways that adults cannot do. The more withdrawn child who finds it hard to participate seems to gain from the more aggressive child courage to begin to move out. The child who wants more than his share of turns, who finds it hard not to have the first turn or to wait while others have a turn, gets his behavior modified with being helped to wait for others. The child who seems to be denying the stuttering, even though it is severe, is helped by the child who can say easily, "That was pretty easy," or "I surely got stuck that time." The responses of other children to a child's success seem to "get through" to the child in their own special way.

When the therapist implements attitudes of acceptance of the children, including the stuttering, provides for freedom within the limits of group behavior and respects each child with his own uniqueness, the children pick up these attitudes toward themselves and each other. In this context the experience of the part of themselves which is speech in relation to the experience of being part of a group seems to serve an important function for the child who stutters.

Therapy for Parents

Therapy for parents is conceived as an integral part of therapy for the child who stutters. In practice, therapy has involved mothers primarily, although on occasion fathers have attended regular group meetings, and they have often come in for specially arranged appointments. The parent therapy group meets one hour each day while the children are in the therapy session. Individual appointments are scheduled during the second hour that the child is attending the clinic. Limitations of clinic staff time may reduce these individual appointments to a minimum, although the value of a combination of group and individual experience is recognized for parents as well as children. Where individual therapy for a particular parent has seemed especially important, referral is made to the University psychological clinic where regular individual time can be provided. This discussion will concern group therapy for parents, since this has regularly been made available.

When a child is brought for the original diagnostic interview the treatment plan is explained to parents as including the mother's attendance with the child. If the mother's attendance is impossible, the child may be taken and individual arrangements are made with parents. With such advance planning, however, most mothers can arrange to attend. Some have taken leaves-of-absence from work or arranged for baby sitters. Experience has indicated that families feel they also need help, respond to the importance of their being involved in the child's therapy, and accept such arrangements as part of their planning for therapy.

The content of therapy for parents without any clear cut division of time follows that of therapy for children; that is, the parent's experience of himself as a whole and the experience of that part which relates specifically to the child's speech. That parents need experience which helps with their own self-affirmation and self-actualization as a total functioning person is recognized in the literature from child guidance clinics or wherever helping relationships have been directed to parents specifically. Parents of children who stutter also need information and help specific to the child's speech.

Parents of children who stutter need help not because they necessarily are particularly neurotic people, but they are confronting a particular problem with their child in speech, and this seems a potent agent for attacking their sense of self. It announces itself to the world in a way in which many other problems they face do not. Although all the parents enrolled in a group may not have children who stutter, they all have a child with some kind of speech problem, and this gives a common ground which seems to promote sharing of common problems. One mother of a child who stuttered said one day to a mother whose child had a cleft palate, "You're lucky in some ways. At least you have something you couldn't help that *caused* your child's speech problem and I have to feel responsible for mine." The other mother said she'd never thought of it like that because she had kept thinking what she might have done or not done which caused the child to be born that way. After some discussion, they both agreed that for them feeling "responsible" was the hardest part to bear. Their resentment, powerlessness, shame, and a wish for a magic cure are common themes.

Parents often comment toward the end of a session that they can't talk to their friends at home like they talk at the clinic because their friends' children all seem so perfect. The majority of the discussions, however, usually have been on topics common to any mothers. Mothers who work outside the home and those who don't discuss advantages annd disadvantages of both. Such topics as their needs for something to nourish them as people apart from being mothers and their feelings that they do all the giving in the family are common. Reports from mothers of more positive feelings about their functioning as mothers and as persons have also indicated that pressures on the child resulting from the mother's concern are reduced.

Much of the content of the group discussion relates specifically to the child's speech. Such questions as, "Is stuttering inherited?", "Will my younger child learn stuttering from his older brother?" "Does he stutter because he can think faster than he can talk?" seem to indicate the need for giving the best information our field has to offer. Parents are helped with ways of simplifying at least some communicative situations for the child at home. They may observe a therapist in an activity designed for this purpose. This gives the mother something valid and appropriate which she can do and seems to make it easier for her to follow the therapist's suggestion that she discontinue such practices as stopping the child when he stutters and having him start over or nagging him to slow down.

Therapy for parents of children who stutter is considered to be an important correlate to therapy for the child. It provides help for the parent in coping with her life as a whole and in coping with her child's speech. Perhaps no less important is that her involvement in and importance to the treatment program does not surrogate her primary role in the significant happenings of her child's life.

Summary

A concept of therapy for adults, children and parents in terms of the individual's experiences of self has been presented. Attention has been paid to the role of the therapist in creating a therapeutic relationship in which the clinical activities gain meaning. The therapeutic relationship is based on assumptions that each individual has intrinsic worth and an inherent drive toward growth. It is the task of therapy to provide an environment of warmth, acceptance and opportunity for success in which the individual may integrate his experiences into his self-structure.

References

1. Axline, V. M.: *Play Therapy*. Boston, Houghton-Mifflin Co., 1947.
2. Backus, O.: Group structure in speech therapy, in Travis, L., ed.: *Handbook of Speech Pathology*. New York, Appleton-Century-Croft, 1957.
3. Backus, O. and Beasley, J.: *Speech Therapy with Children*. Boston, Houghton-Mifflin Co., 1951.

4. Bloodstein, O.: Stuttering as an anticipatory struggle reaction, in Eisenson, J., ed.: *Stuttering: A Symposium.* New York, Harper and Brothers, 1958.

4a. Clark, R. and Fitzpatrick, J.: The Use of Self-concept as an adjunct to diagnosis and psychotherapy, in Barbara, D., ed.: *The Psychotherapy of Stuttering.* Springfield, Illinois, Charles C Thomas, 1962.

5. Dorfman, E.: Play therapy, in Rogers, C.: *Client-Centered Therapy.* Boston, Houghton-Mifflin Co., 1951.

6. Eisenson, J.: A perseverative theory of stuttering, in Eisenson, J., ed.: *Stuttering: A Symposium.* New York, Harper and Brothers, 1958.

7. Glauber, I. P.: The psychoanalysis of stuttering, in Eisenson, J., ed.: *Stuttering: A Symposium.* New York, Harper and Brothers, 1958.

8. Goldstein, K.: *Human Nature in the Light of Psychopathology.* Cambridge, Harvard University Press, 1940.

9. Hall, C. S. and Lindzey, G.: *Theories of Personality.* New York, John Wiley and Sons, 1957.

10. Horney, K.: *Neurotic Personality of our Times.* New York, Norton, 1937.

11. Johnson, W.: Perceptual and evaluational factors in stuttering, in Travis, L., ed.: *Handbook of Speech Pathology.* New York, Appleton-Century-Croft, 1957.

12. Lewin, K.: *Field Theory in Social Science.* Cartwright, D., ed., New York, Harper, 1951.

13. Martin, E.: Client-centered therapy as a theoretical orientation for speech therapy. *Asha, 5:* 576, 1963.

14. Moreno, J. L.: *Psychodrama.* Beacon, New York, Beacon House, 1959.

14a. Murphy, A. and Fitzsimons, R.: *Stuttering and Personality Dynamics.* New York, Ronald Press, 1960.

15. Rogers, C. R.: *Client-Centered Therapy.* Boston, Houghton-Mifflin, 1951.

15a. Shearer, W.: A theoretical consideration of the self-concept and body image in stuttering therapy. *ASHA, 3:* 115, 1961.

16. Sheehan, J.: Conflict theory of stuttering, in Eisenson, J., ed.: *Stuttering: A Symposium.* New York, Harper and Brothers, 1958.

17. Snygg, D. and Combs, A. W.: *Individual Behavior.* New York, Harper and Brothers, 1949.

18. Sullivan, H. S.: *The Interpersonal Theory of Psychiatry.* New York, Norton, 1953.

19. Tillich, P.: *The Courage To Be*. New York, Charles Scribner's Sons, 1957.
20. Van Riper, C.: Symptomatic therapy for stuttering, in Travis, L., ed.: *Handbook of Speech Pathology*. New York, Appleton-Century-Croft, 1957.
21. West, R.: An agnostic's speculations about stuttering, in Eisenson, J., ed.: *Stuttering: A Symposium*. New York, Harper and Brothers, 1958.
22. Williams, D.: A point of view about stuttering. *J. Speech Hearing Dis., 22:* 390, 1957.
23. Wyatt, G.: Stuttering in pre-school children: a disorder of language learning. Unpublished material.

7

Alterations in Self-Concept: A Barometer of Progress in Individuals Undergoing Therapy for Stuttering

Ruth Millburn Clark, Ph.D.
Frederick Pemberton Murray, M.A.

Vorchristliche Zeit

20. Jahrhundert

Aus der ersten Zeit des mittleren altägyptischen Reiches (ab 2000 v. Chr.) läßt sich auf dem Papyrus Golenischeff Z. 17 („Schiffbrüchiger") ein Verbum ⁓ 𓈖𓂋𓈖𓂋 𓁿 *nitit* „z ö g e r n d sprechen", „stottern" o. ä. belegen. *nitit* ist nur eine graphische Radikallesung der Ägyptologen und stellt eine sogenannte Niphal-Bildung von einem reduplizierten Verbalstamm √ ῾t ῾t dar. Seinem Sinn nach geht es auf eine retardierende Bewegung des Gehens zurück, übertragen auf den „Gang" der Rede mit dem Vehikel der Zunge, was also ursprünglich ein Bild vom zaghaft retardierenden Treten der Beine gewesen war, wurde bildhaft auf die „Gang"-Bewegung der Zunge übertragen. Ausdrücklich ergibt sich aus dem Zusammenhang in der oben zitierten Belegstelle, daß es sich um die Art zu reden bei einem Menschen handelt, der aus tiefer Angstdepression sein „Herz" nicht „in der Hand" hat. Wohl der älteste Beleg für eine Sprachstörung. (2)

Translation*

Pre-christian Era 20th Century (B. C.)

During the first part of the middle of the ancient Egyptian Empire (Circa 2,000 years before Christ), there existed on the papyrus Golinischeff Z. 17 ("The Shipwrecked"), a verb:

〜〜〜 ⌇ ⌒ ⌇ ⌒ 🐦   *nitit* "to talk hesitantly," "to stutter."

Nitit is a graphic radical reading of the Egyptiologists and represents a so-called Niphil-form of a reduplicated verbal root √ 't 't. Its basic sense refers to a retarding movement of the walking mechanism, in a figurative sense it refers to the "gait" of talking with the vehicle of the tongue. What was originally a picture of the reluctant retarded stepping of the legs, was figuratively applied to the stepping (walking) movements of the tongue. The context of the above quotation (see the picture) expresses very definitely that it deals with an individual, who because of deep fear-depression, does not have "his heart in his hands." This may be the oldest evidence of a speech defect.

Stuttering seems to have been plaguing humanity for a long, long time. Man has been writing about the problem and seeking a solution to it for some four thousand years and, still, all parts of the puzzle have not as yet been assembled. Winston Churchill once referred to the Soviet Union as "An enigma inside a riddle wrapped in a mystery." This same quotation could surely be applied to stuttering.

In trying to understand this enigma of stuttering and to perceive some of the mysteries concerning it, a voluminous amount of speculation, writing and research has taken place. In the literature relating to stuttering frequent reference has recently been made to the body image or self-concept that stutterers have about themselves.

Self-concept is the mental representation an individual has of his own body or "self." Emotional experiences, fantasies, postural changes and internal sensations, contact with people and objects, successes and failures all unite in forming an individual's self concept. "It includes both the conscious and unconscious attitudes, memories, feelings, and fairly stable characteristics that one has

---

*Courtesy Dr. G. H. Breckwoldt, Saint Louis University, Saint Louis, Missouri.

regarding himself and his place in society. It is an individual's re-action to his bodily and mental processes" (4, p. 164).

According to Schilder (14) human beings have strong emotions concerning their own bodies, and there exists a very close relation-ship between the perceptive (afferent-impressive) side of one's psychic life and the motor (efferent-expressive) activities. Pertin-ent to the feedback that the stutterer receives from the peripheral organs of speech is the relationship that Schilder reported relative to the most sensitive zones of the body. He indicated these zones as being near the openings of the body and approximately one centimeter inside the body. The act of speaking probably involves changes in pressure and tension to more of these sensitive areas than most other physical acts. The palate, ears, nose and mouth are all stimulated during speech. The overactivity of the peripheral speech organs in a stuttering block will have a decided effect on the emotions of the stutterer and in turn the resultant self-concept.

Changing the stutterer's self-concept concerning speech and his feelings about it constitutes a vital part of the therapeutic program. According to leading authorities, "with many people who stutter, a major part of their problem seems to involve a disturbed concept of themselves as being different from other people" (16, p.p. 27-28).

Many leading psychologists indicate that if therapy is to be effective, there is a definite need for more understanding of the private world of the individual. Since a person unconsciously re-veals many things about his self-concept through projective tests, they have proven to be of value. Following are some techniques that are used to gain insight into an individual's self-concept or to ascertain how he "perceives, conceives and evaluates" his world: Diagnostic Interest Blanks, Goodenough Draw-A-Man Test, Mach-over Draw-A-Person Investigations, doll play, finger painting, pup-pet therapy, House-Tree-Person (H-T-P) test, Make a Picture Story (MAPS) test, Psychodrama, Rorschach Test, Szondi Test, Thematic Apperception Test (TAT), Children's Apperception Test (CAT), Mosaic Test, Word Association Tests, Self Ratings, Autobiography, Q-sort technique, Stuttering Behavior Analysis and the Who Are You (W-A-Y) test. The following discussion is con-cerned with the use of the last four techniques in ascertaining changes in the self-concept of individuals who stutter.

W - A - Y Technique

Bugental and Zelen, (1) stimulated by Raimy's (12) research, designed the "W-A-Y" or "Who Are You?" approach to the study of self-concept. They experimented with various types of interview techniques and found the W-A-Y question to be the most revealing of self-concept trends. The subject is asked to give three answers to the question, "Who are you?" The reply may be words, phrases, or anything that satisfies the individual that each response has answered the question. The subject is allowed to structure his responses along lines most meaningfully related to his current situation and most expressive of his own needs. The question allows a free field for response and yet is sufficiently structured to allow statistical analysis.

The following categories were established statistically for the analysis of the data:

1. Name.
2. Personal pronoun.
3. Nonindividualized reference.
4. Sex.
5. Age.
6. Occupation.
7. Family status.
8. Social status.
9. Neutral descriptive references.
10. Affectively tone reference.
11. Miscellaneous (1).

The designers of the W-A-Y technique felt that if offered a great deal in exploring the self-concept of individuals. They were impressed with the functionality and theoretical relevance of the method.

Zelen, Sheehan and Bugental used the W-A-Y technique with thirty stutterers and then compared the self-perceptions of this experimental group with a control group of 160 normal speakers. Results of the study were in agreement with the findings of other research that positive feelings increase and negative feelings decrease with successful psychotherapy. They concluded that:

The use of the W-A-Y technique for predicting the stutterer's response to treatment is suggested by the observed tendency of the eventually successful patients to start therapy with fewer negative self-percepts (19, p. 72).

Parks (11) used an extension of the W-A-Y technique. Seven more questions similar in structure and purpose were added to the original W-A-Y question. The questionnaire items and instructions to the subjects were as follows:

> In the questionnaire that I have given you, you will find a series of eight questions. Three answer spaces are supplied for each question. You are simply to read the question, then give three answers. The three answers may be anything you want them to be—they may be words, phrases, sentences or anything at all, so long as you are satisfied that each one answers the question (11 p. 11).

1. Who are you?

    _____

    _____

    _____

2. What is your goal?

    _____

    _____

    _____

3. What do you expect you will be?

    _____

    _____

    _____

4. What is life?

    _____

    _____

    _____

5. What is the most unpleasant thing you can think of?

    _____

    _____

    _____

6. What change would you like to make in yourself?

    _____

    _____

    _____

7. What change would you like to make in your everyday world?

    _____

    _____

    _____

8. What is the most satisfactory thing about you?

_____

_____

_____

The three responses lead the subject to change his set between answers within the question rather than rank the replies. Parks (11) and Bugental (1) feel that this is a fundamental asset of the W-A-Y technique approach.

Parks developed a scoring system on a 1 to 4 point continuum, i.e., "from egoistic, personally focused orientation (1) to altruistic, socially focused orientation (4)" (11 p. 25). The scale included the following, and examples were given for scoring the answers:

1. *Personal* or *egoistic* responses.
2. *Specific* response, referring still to self-orientation, but in a recognizably more objective, less personal manner.
3. *General* response, referring to abstraction and tending more toward group identification.
4. *Social* or *altruistic* response, wherein the identification of self is seen to be *for* the group (11 p. 13).

The investigator felt he had demonstrated that the expanded W-A-Y technique was a productive research approach to the study of self-concept and that the method could be "applied fruitfully to pre- and post-psychotherapy evaluation" (11 p. 28).

Freeman (8) suggested that the use of the W-A-Y technique should be limited to exploratory studies since the results of his research using this method raised the question regarding its reliability.

Since personality is extremely complex and has many facets, and since precise measuring instruments to determine the self-concept of individuals are not as yet "tested and found worthy", perhaps we are justified in using any method that holds out hope of giving us greater insight into the complex personalities of human beings.

Q-Technique

There has been an incessant search for new psychological techniques to help in understanding the personality structure of man. "One of the more promising of these is the Q-technique, a method of intercorrelation of persons developed in England and brought to this country by Stephenson" (7 p. 110). This test attempts to compare an individual's concept of himself with similar self-concepts of others. The subject is asked to describe himself by sorting a series of descriptive statements. It is possible by quantifying these self-descriptions to correlate one person's description of himself with those of others. Through this technique some interesting insights into behavior and personality structure have been obtained. It has "also opened a variety of other areas to more systematic investigation" (7 p. 110).

Q-methodology makes it possible for investigations of a single individual to be undertaken. Most methods require a small number of measurements on a large number of people. Q-methodology requires a large number of measurements on one person or a small group (9).

For a number of years a group at the Counseling Center of the University of Chicago has carried on a "complex and ramified" research program. The Q-technique has been used extensively in many of its research projects. In the preface of the book which co-ordinated the different investigations carried on over a period of several years, the authors made particular mention of "William Stephenson, whose development of the Q-technique supplied us at a most appropriate time with an instrument of great subtlety, stimulating our investigations of areas heretofore beyond our reach" (13 p. VI).

The term *Q-sort* refers to the data gathering procedure used with the Q-technique. The method may be used to investigate any subject for which a special Q-sort has been prepared. Rogers and associates developed their Q-sort to test the self concept of individuals undergoing psychotherapy.

The *Q-adjustment score* was devised to give an external standard of adjustment level. It is based on the Q-sort test, devised by the Rogers group, in which the subject is required to sort a hundred statements into nine piles, putting a prescribed number of cards into each pile, thus making a forced normal distribution. The subject is told to put the cards most descriptive of him at one end and those least descriptive of him at the opposite end. Those about which he is indifferent or undecided are placed around the middle of the distribution. This will produce a distribution as follows:

	"Least Like Me"						"Most Like Me"
Pile No. 0	1	2	3	4	5	6	7	8
No. of Cards 1	4	11	21	26	21	11	4	1

(6, p. 77).

The twenty-six cards in Pile No. 4 are discarded, thus making 74 the highest possible adjustment score. The criterion used to establish the Q-adjustment score and the statements contributing to the negative and positive scores may be found in the book, *Psychotherapy and Personality Change* (13).

The above mentioned Q-sort was the one used with the stutterers herein described. A copy of the Adjustment Score Items (74 Statements) follows:

TABLE I

Adjustment Score Items

Q-Sort Item No.	Statement	Q-Sort Item No.	Statement
	Negative: Contribute to Score if fall on "Unlike Me" Side (0-3)		Positive: Contribute to Score if fall on "Like Me" Side (5-8)
2	I put on a false front.	4	I make strong demands on myself.
6	I often feel humiliated.		
7	I doubt my sexual powers.	5	I often kick myself for the things I do.
13	I have a feeling of hopelessness.		
		9	I have a warm emotional relationship with others.
16	I have few values and standards of my own.		
18	It is difficult to control my aggression.	11	I am responsible for my troubles.
		12	I am a responsible person.
25	I want to give up trying to cope with the world.	15	I can accept most social values and standards.
28	I tend to be on my guard with people who are somewhat more friendly than I had expected.	19	Self control is no problem to me.
		22	I usually like people.
		23	I express my emotions freely.
32	I usually feel driven.	26	I can usually live comfortably with the people around me.
36	I feel helpless.		
38	My decisions are not my own.	27	My hardest battles are with myself.
40	I am a hostile person.		
42	I am disorganized.	29	I am optimistic.
43	I feel apathetic.	33	I am liked by most people who know me.
49	I don't trust my emotions.		
50	It's pretty tough to be me.	35	I am sexually attractive.

TABLE I — (Continued)

Adjustment Score Items

Q-Sort Item No.	Statement	Q-Sort Item No.	Statement
	Negative: Contribute to Score if fall on "Unlike Me" Side (0-3)		Positive: Contribute to Score if fall on "Like Me" Side (5-8)
52	I have the feeling that I am just not facing things.	37	I can usually make up my mind and stick to it.
54	I try not to think about my problems.	41	I am contented.
56	I am shy.	44	I am poised.
59	I am no one. Nothing seems to be me.	47	I am impulsive.
62	I despise myself.	51	I am a rational person.
64	I shrink from facing a crisis or difficulty.	53	I am tolerant.
65	I just don't respect myself.	55	I have an attractive personality.
69	I am afraid of a full-fledged disagreement with a person.	61	I am ambitious.
70	I can't seem to make up my mind one way or another.	63	I have initiative.
71	I am confused.	67	I take a positive attitude toward myself.
73	I am a failure.	68	I am assertive.
76	I am afraid of sex.	72	I am satisfied with myself.
77	I have a horror of failing in anything I want to accomplish.	74	I am likable.
83	I really am disturbed.	75	My personality is attractive to the opposite sex.
84	All you have to do is just insist with me, and I give in.	78	I am relaxed, and nothing bothers me.
85	I feel insecure within myself.	79	I am a hard worker.
86	I have to protect myself with excuses, with rationalizing.	80	I feel emotionally mature.
90	I feel hopeless.	88	I am intelligent.
95	I am unreliable.	91	I am self-reliant.
99	I am worthless.	94	I am different from others.
100	I dislike my own sexuality.	96	I understand myself.
		97	I am a good mixer.
		98	I feel adequate.

(6, p. 79).

Stuttering Behavior Analysis

A Stuttering Behavior Analysis Chart (3) can be used to show changes in self-concept as therapy progresses and also to compare an individual's evaluation of his speech with the appraisal given by his associates.

Until objectivity has advanced sufficiently to use the behavior analysis in group situations, it can be used individually. The person evaluates his speech and explains the reasons for the marks given. As therapy progresses, other evaluations are made on the same chart so progress and change may be noted.

All speech defectives present an individual problem, but most stutterers also present common problems. Numerous authorities agree that group work for stutterers is effective for many purposes such as sharing experiences, information and feelings, and providing natural audience situations for practice. This development of group morale does much to enhance the motivations of the individual members.

For group situations the Stuttering Behavior Analysis Chart is a useful therapeutic device. As indicated on the following chart, each member of the group is assigned a color. After oral reports are given, each participant puts a mark in his color on the respective line of the chart, thus indicating his analysis of his performance in all of the categories. The person doing the rating and the members of the group then discuss the reasons for the marks given and any changes or alteration in speaking that are desirable.

Further use can be made of the chart by having each individual

Stuttering Behavior Analysis

	Unusual				*Normal*
I. *Visible Aspects*	1	2	3	4	5
a. Forcing					
b. Grimaces					
II. *Audible Aspects*					
a. Pitch					
b. Loudness (Intensity)					
c. Voice quality					
d. Rate-rhythm					
III. *Emotional Aspects*					
a. Embarrassment and shame					
b. Avoidance (words and situations)					
c. Fears					

Assign each person in class a color: Use different symbol for each evaluation:

Joan—Purple	First Evaluation—Circle ●
John—Green	Second Evaluation—Square ■
Bill—Blue	Third Evaluation—Star ★
Joe—Red	Fourth Evaluation—Triangle ▲
George—Yellow	

in the group rate everyone else in the group and explain why the ratings were given.

The chart can also provide a means of objectively measuring improvement in the characteristics listed. That is, the first Analysis Chart can be filed after it has been marked and the ratings discussed. At the end of the term the individual can be graded on another chart and the two profiles compared.

One caution should be noted: this chart should probably not be employed with a group in the beginning of therapy, but rather after the individuals have gained some insight into their problems and have achieved a certain amount of objectivity.

Autobiography

A valuable source of information to ascertain an individual's conception of himself is the autobiography. According to Strang the autobiography affords great potential for studying individuals. She said that if one were limited to using only two of all the techniques available to the teacher for evaluating a person, "observation and the autobiography would probably give the best understanding of the individual's behavior and of his unique ways of viewing and interpreting his world" (17 pp. 87-88).

Numerous references could be cited that attest to the value of autobiography—among them Snygg and Combs (15), who agree that it is a valuable instrument in studying personality.

From a research conducted by Curtis, he concluded that justification for using the autobiography as a measure of personality was founded on the following:

> 1) Consistency of personality descriptions in autobiography is higher than has been suspected previously, and 2) subjects may admit certain "weaknesses" of their personalities, that is, acknowledge what they perceive as limitations of the self, with greater facility when writing an autobiography than in subsequent self-evaluations such as questionnaires and similar personality measuring devices (5 p. 5 of abstract of dissertation).

Having the individual who stutters write his personal history can be enlightening in many instances. From the written narrative much is revealed about his feelings toward himself and his speech problem, as well as about his associates and his past and present environments. The autobiography provides insight into how he perceives himself and his world, as well as his role in it. The writer divulges a great deal by his omissions, under-evaluations, or emphasis on certain periods or points in his history. Many times facts and attitudes are revealed in writing that would not be unveiled in the oral interview. "In the preparation of such a document there is also bound to be conscious and unconscious selection of items. Inevitably topics will be omitted which you might want to know about" (10 p. 24).

As with many projective techniques, the autobiography has a therapeutic as well as a diagnostic value. Frequently the individual who has had therapy is able to write a more comprehensive and insightful report and, through it, disclose more adequately his self-concept. More pertinent material is usually brought forth if the person is properly prepared for the assignment and if an outline, such as the following one, is given to him and thoroughly discussed:

Outline for an Autobiography of Student's Speech History

I. Personal History:
1. Number of brothers and sisters.
2. Subject's rank in order of birth.
3. Handedness. Which hand do you use? Has your handedness ever been changed?
4. Any twins in the family.
5. Anyone else in the family or any relatives that stutter?
6. Hobbies and interests.
7. Languages spoken in the home.
8. In silent reading do you consider yourself slow, rapid, average?
9. Are you awkward, clumsy, rhythmic, graceful?
10. Are your parents alive and living together? If not—explain status.

II. Health History:
1. Serious illness.
2. Mannerisms and nervous disturbances such as: thumbsucking, nailbiting, sleeplessness, nightmares, twitching, etc.
3. Physical injuries.
4. Fears
5. Disposition: happy, sad, changeable, moody, sullen, quiet, friendly, quarrelsome, obstinate, suggestible, jealous, affectionate, adaptable, resentful.

6. Have yon now or ever had any allergies? If so, what and when?
7. Have you now or ever had any respitory difficulties, such as asthma? If so, what and when?

III. *Speech History*:

1. When did you begin to talk?
2. When did your stuttering begin?
3. Does your stuttering run in cycles; that is, is it better at times? When? Is it worse at times? When?
4. When did you become conscious of stuttering?
5. Recount a number of embarrassing situations you have been in because of your stuttering.
6. What was the family attitude toward you? Over-indulgent; indifferent; tendency to shield you and take your part; tendency to be cruel and to laugh and make fun of you?
7. What is your attitude toward your stuttering?
   a. Is it an objective, matter-of-fact, realistic point of view?
   b. Do you think of it critically and constructively?
   c. Can you talk about it unemotionally?
   d. Are you over-sensitive about your stuttering?
   e. Do you exaggerate the handicap of stuttering?
   f. Do you enjoy being with people or do you avoid them?
   g. Do you accuse other people of making fun of you because of your stuttering?
8. Have you done anything yourself to improve your speech? If so, what?
9. What helps you the most to reduce your stuttering spasms?
10. Are some sounds more difficult for you than others? Which ones?
11. Over the past three years has your stuttering become worse, better or stayed the same?
12. Do you stutter when you talk to yourself; your pets; younger or older people; people of the same sex or opposite sex.
13. With what people and under what conditions is your stuttering the worst?
14. With what people and under what conditions is your speech the best?
15. What do you think caused your stuttering?
16. Can you predict occurrence of your stuttering?
17. Can you visualize yourself as a normal speaker?
18. Is there anything else about your speech you consider interesting?

IV. Speech Therapy
　　1. Have you had speech therapy? If so, where? For how long?
　　2. Briefly describe the treatment.
　　3. Were you receptive to the ideas in therapy?
　　4. Did you progress? In what ways? Speech? Attitudes?
　　5. What was your original goal in speech therapy?
　　6. What are your present speech goals?
　　7. Do you consider yourself a treatment success? Explain.

Results and Evaluations

As everyone in the field of Speech Pathology knows, the literature covering the general topic of stuttering is voluminous. In spite of this, very few writers have approached the problem from the point of view of self-concept as the major emphasis in comprehending and working with the stutterer.

Freeman said, "To understand the stutterer as an individual, or as a client undergoing therapy, it is of utmost importance to view him in relation to how he thinks, feels, acts, and perceives his environment; likewise, how the environmental sources interact upon him" (8 p. 31).

More and more authorities are sensing that to effectively treat an individual who stutters, one must consider, evaluate and work with his self-concept. Raimy (12) believes that changes in self-concept and resultant personality reorganization can be detected by measuring changes in a client's attitude toward himself. The present study does not evaluate changes in the self-concept of any one individual as he progresses in therapy, but rather gives the self-concept of three different individuals as shown by the four previously-discussed instruments. These three subjects received different amounts of therapy.

These subjects were all males enrolled in the Adult Stutterer's Therapy Group at the University of Denver Speech, Hearing and Language Clinic. This group met weekly for one and one-half hours. Subject Number I, Claude, was new in therapy. Subject Number II, Mark, had been with the group for twenty meetings. Victor, the last case presented, had had extensive therapy for a number of years.

Subject I:

Claude, at the time he took the tests, had been with the group for three sessions only. Although he was the youngest member of the group, he was an apt subject because of his willingness to cooperate and because of his ability to express himself both in writing and in speaking, despite frequent clonic and tonic blocks.

W-A-Y TEST

Average Answer Score—1.7: This indicated a marked tendency toward personal and egoistic responses. Many of his answers showed preoccupation with self and little concern about society in general. Regarding life, he stated that it was a mess and consisted of a small circle. His impression was that he was in the middle of this circle and its boundaries were very constricting.

Q-SORT TEST

Q-adjustment Score—55: This score can be interpreted as meaning that the subject tended toward positive self-evaluation, although the possibility of this being exaggerated because of his "idealized self-image" was great. He seemed to lack a realistic, truthful, conception of himself. In spite of the fact that he was rendered almost speechless many times because of his stuttering blocks, in sorting the statements he indicated that he did not feel humiliated, nor shy, nor helpless in any way. Results of the two succeeding tests, as well as the therapist's evaluation, substantiated the hypothesis as presented below.

STUTTERING BEHAVIOR ANALYSIS

A wide disparity of scores between Claude's self-rating and the rating of his performance by the other members of the group gave evidence of his over-estimated self-evaluation. It is well known that even very severe stutterers make every attempt to cover up as many facts of their problem as possible. In this case, the self-ratings of the overt symptom, visible aspects, were in line with the evaluations of the other members of the group. However, it is interesting to note that on matters concerning the audible and emotional aspects of his speech, he gave himself a normal score while the other members of the group did not support this rating (see Figure 2).

This suggested that he was not being realistic about his speech problem. The other members of the group felt in both of these aspects that his speech was unusual. In no instance did they rate him above average, and half of the audible scores were evaluated at the lowest level. He rated himself as normal in every category except rhythm; in this aspect he scored himself as average.

An interpretation of this might be that a large part of his problem results from a role conflict. This probably results from his refusal to admit to himself that he is a severe stutterer. He therefore tries to play the role of a fluent speaker. If this thesis is correct, therapy should be structured along the lines of psychotherapy enabling this faulty self-concept to be replaced by a more realistic one. It appeared that this conflict arose because of his lack of objectivity toward his problem.

Stuttering Behavior Analysis

	Unusual				Normal
I. *Visible Aspects*	1	2	3	4	5
a. Forcing	X	√ O			
b. Grimaces	X	O	√		
II. *Audible Aspects*					
a. Pitch	O			X	√
b. Loudness (Intensity)			O	X	√
c. Voice Quality	O	X			√
d. Rate-rhythm	X	O	√		
III. *Emotional Aspects*					
a. Embarrassment and Shame			O	X	√
b. Avoidance (Words and Situations)			X	O	√
c. Fears			O	X	√

Figure 2

Subject I — Claude

√ = Self Evaluation
X = Therapist's Evaluation
O = Group's Evaluation

AUTOBIOGRAPHY

Claude gave the following interesting and perhaps significant statements in his self-history:

My grandfather on my father's side stuttered and my brother starts to stutter when he gets excited . . . I bite my nails off and on. I've had my arm broken and I've had a concussion. I don't seem to have any fears . . . I have hay-fever in the spring and fall . . . I first began to stutter at three and one-half years old and have stuttered ever since . . . I can't remember any embarrassing situations at all . . . I enjoy talking to other people . . . I cannot predict when I will stutter. I always visualize myself as a normal speaker.

Claude's autobiography substantiated many of the foregoing evaluations. His concept of himself as a normal speaker is confirmed by his Stuttering Behavior Analysis. Out of nine sub-areas, he evaluated himself as normal in six of them. The discrepancy between his evaluation and that of the other members of the group was cited earlier.

Contrary to Claude's stated experience, it is rare to find a severe stutterer who is unable to predict any of his blocks or who cannot recall any embarrassing situations connected with his stuttering.

The extremely sharp contrast between the actual facts and Claude's visualization of himself as a normal speaker points to the importance of therapy in helping him establish a more accurate representation of himself. His apparent blindness to his problem and his unrealistic attitude regarding it must be recognized and faced squarely by him before he can attain any substantial progress in overcoming his handicap.

EVALUATION BY THE THERAPIST

Claude is still quite young but seems to have a good rational mind which on the surface gives him a rather satisfactory appearance of adjustment. His stuttering is very severe with many breathy intakes, bounces, prolongations, etc. His attitude is one of egocentricity when he says he enjoys speaking to others at all times, for his behavior in therapy is not in agreement with his expressed attitudes. Generally, he speaks only when called upon.

Subject II:

Mark, subject II, had attended therapy sessions for almost six months when his tests were taken. Although his fluency was quite adequate in ordinary situations, he stuttered noticeably under communicative stress, the stuttering being characterized by sudden oscillations enforced by tension. This man was vividly aware of his stuttering and had, for years, been trying to find a quick solution to overcome it. Although only a few years past college age, he was mature in many ways, especially regarding cultural things. Mark was verbal and expressed himself frequently at the therapy sessions. He presented anxiety and concern over the interruptions that occurred in his speech, but declared that these feelings were beginning to diminish. He attributed this to some changes that were developing in his attitudes.

W-A-Y TEST

Average Answer Score—2.3: This score would indicate that the subject had a moderate amount of self-concern. However, this is probably elevated because of his philosophical and altruistic goals and does not accurately portray the concern he had about his speech problem. This is borne out by the following statement: "I would like to be able to express myself freely without anguish." In another section, he stated that he was extremely uncomfortable when he was unable "to express to others, in decent language, what I want to say."

At one point in the test he revealed that his ultimate goal was to help others realize their potentialities. Thus, it was clear that Mark had worthwhile goals, but he also realized that in order to reach them he would have to achieve significantly more skill communicationwise to be able to relate to others more effectively.

Q-SORT TEST

Q-adjustment Score—41: This revealed that Mark's self-concept, as shown by this test, was just slightly above average. An indication of this was his willingness to assume responsibility for his troubles and his feeling that he was not a hostile individual. He also indicated that he had warm relationships with others.

In spite of this average personality adjustment, he disclosed there were many situations which were threatening to him. On the whole, many of the statements he selected on the test revealed that he believed he had the ability to improve and that he held high hopes for the future.

The results of the Q-sort Test manifested that his selection of statements corresponded rather closely with those aspects of his personality which were perceived in social situations.

STUTTERING BEHAVIOR ANALYSIS

On the whole, the evaluations by the subject, the therapist, and the group were pretty much in harmony. All three of these ratings were within one step of each other, except, for pitch and rhythm under the Audible Aspects. The discrepancy was greatest with respect to rhythm. In this category the subject ranked himself toward the unusual end of the continuum, while the group felt that his rhythm was normal. The same thing occurred where pitch was concerned. The therapist felt his pitch was normal, while the subject and the group felt it was at the midpoint between the unusual and normal. However, on the whole, the differences were not great. This showed that Mark's self-evaluations were in line with the actual situation as far as his stuttering behavior analysis was concerned.

This variation in evaluation of pitch and rhythm might have occurred because Mark said fast speech often helped him to "glide past" stuttering blocks. Since many members of the group presented slow, labored speech, due to their stuttering, the group tended to feel that Mark's fast, rapid rate was more normal.

In discussing the emotional aspects of speech, this subject said that his embarrassment and shame had diminished since he began therapy. He indicated that had the tests been given a few months earlier, he would have rated himself more toward the unusual end of the scale in many areas (see Figure 3).

AUTOBIOGRAPHY

Mark is one of twelve children. A brother, who died in his youth, was the only other member of the family who stuttered. Evidence of some bilingual conflicts in the home were shown in the history.

An exploration of Mark's health history shows nothing whatsoever to be significant in this area. In fact, he has enjoyed extremely good health. He related that "fear states" often have caused him temporary unpleasant sensations.

Speech seemed to have followed a normal sequence of development until Mark was seven years of age. At that time he started to stutter. He had more difficulty in the school situation than in the home. He related being put under obligation to speak in competitive circumstances, and he felt that these situations caused the speech difficulty to flourish. Embarrassment grew rapidly, and by the time he was in high school his stuttering had become fortified with many emotional components. For years he felt that his speech problem was a great liability and was holding him back from success in many situations.

In his autobiography Mark indicated that he considered his stuttering undesirable, but he felt he was making a more realistic re-appraisal of it. For example, he stated that he could now talk about stuttering without "going to pieces." He indicated that voluntary stuttering had helped him confront, alter, and accept his speech difficulty. In the past Mark had great resistance to "stuttering on purpose," but later realized if he accepted and practiced the technique wholeheartedly, it would help him achieve the genuine self-pride that he desired so much. He was aware that in the past his goals had been set too high.

About three years ago Mark undertook one semester of therapy in another institution, using hypnosis as its basis. He indicated that the aim was to reduce nervous tension as well as to solve the stuttering. He was benefitted, at least temporarily, in both of these aspects, but he soon lapsed back into his old patterns. Until recently, his goal was complete fluency of speech. However, during therapy he became more realistic in this regard and said he wished "to become so proficient in *stuttering adequately* that it will hardly be noticeable to the listener.'

EVALUATION BY THE THERAPIST

Mark's speech is quite rapid. His stuttering is usually mild except in emotionally surcharged situations. He states that it used to be worse. Mark seems to have a fairly good overall adjustment but is rather quiet until he feels he knows you. He thinks that his drawbacks are largely speech patterns rather than psychological factors within himself.

Subject III:

Victor, the oldest of the three subjects discussed in this chapter, had been exposed to more speech therapy than the other two. He had also had several years of teaching experience. Although formerly a severe stutterer, his speech had improved sufficiently to enable him to maintain his position as a teacher.

W-A-Y TEST

Average Answer Score—2.9: This indicated that the subject gave answers tending toward group identification. However, these were mixed in with some subjective responses, as well as with some statements concerning the good of mankind. He mentioned as one of his goals that of wanting to bring peace to humanity and of serving mankind. Stuttering was mentioned only once during his test. The philosophical and altruistic replies outnumbered the personal and egoistic items.

Q-SORT TEST

Q-adjustment Score—49: A relatively positive self-evaluation was shown by his score. For example, the statements about being ambitious, having initiative, feeling responsible, and making strong demands on himself were all put in the piles representing items "Most Like Me."

On the negative side, or in the piles indicating "Least Like Me," he put statements such as the following: "I am a failure, I feel helpless, I am worthless."

A probable interpretation of this might be that Victor had a sufficient amount of ego-integration to maintain his present fluency, and in all likelihood, to further improve his speech.

STUTTERING BEHAVIOR ANALYSIS

The self concept of Victor seemed to be realistic according to the results of the Stuttering Behavior Analysis.

The predominant feature of this chart was the high degree of correlation shown between the subject's own self-evaluation, and the evaluation of the group. This probably indicated that Victor's stuttering had improved sufficiently so that his speech was no longer a serious handicap to him and that most of the time others considered it normal.

A feasible interpretation of this might be that the handicapping aspects of the problem had been overcome. It also implied that a realistic attitude, one that did not apparently call for defending whatever stuttering spasms remained, had been developed. Most authorities agree that when these objectives have been attained, a practical solution to stuttering has been achieved and it is no longer a hindrance (see Figure 4).

Stuttering Behavior Analysis

	Unusual 1	2	3	4	Normal 5
I. Visible Aspects					
a. Forcing				√XO	
b. Grimaces			XO	√	
II. Audible Aspects					
a. Pitch			√O		X
b. Loudness (Intensity)			√	XO	
c. Voice Quality			√O	X	
d. Rate-rhythm		√	X		O
III. Emotional Aspects					
a. Embarrassment and Shame			X	√O	
b. Avoidance (Words and Situations)				√X	O
c. Fears				√X	O

Figure 3

Subject II — Mark

√ = Self Evaluation
X = Therapist's Evaluation
O = Group's Evaluation

Stuttering Behavior Analysis

	Unusual 1	2	3	4	Normal 5
I. Visible Aspects					
a. Forcing				√X	O
b. Grimaces					√XO
II. Audible Aspects					
a. Pitch					√XO
b. Loudness (Intensity)				O	√X
c. Voice Quality					√XO
d. Rate-rhythm				√XO	
III. Emotional Aspects					
a. Embarrassment and Shame					√XO
b. Avoidance (Words and Situations)				√X	O
c. Fears				X	√O

Figure 4

Subject III — Victor

√ = Self Evaluation
X = Therapist's Evaluation
O = Group's Evaluation

AUTOBIOGRAPHY

Victor said his stuttering began very suddenly after a severe nosebleed, followed by a long, tiring auto trip. In his autobiography he stated "speech that was fluent one night was totally disorganized and unintelligible the following morning." Since he has been working on his speech, he has become convinced that "the stuttering originally arose because of damage to the nervous system."

There was much evidence in his autobiography which pointed to a poor handling of his stuttering problem, especially from the mental hygiene point of view. Victor apparently was made to feel that, in the family circle, stuttering was something to be hidden, concealed, and not discussed. This, together with elementary school speech therapy which aimed at the prevention of the occurrence of stuttering, merely set the pattern for the rapid accumulation of devastating emotional complications. He had accepted possible labeling of the condition, along with other social factors, as merely precipitators that further aggravated the probable neurological deficit.

Victor reported that his high school days were a nightmare from the standpoint of speech. He received no speech help whatsoever at this time, and he found that his fears of stuttering were spreading like "wildfire." Oral recitations and telephoning caused him to block completely. Although his hope had been to go through college and to become a teacher, he felt his stuttering was so severe that he must give up this goal and enter a "non-speaking occupation."

After Victor graduated from high school, he learned about speech clinics connected with universities where research on the stuttering problem was being carried on and where he could receive therapy. Immediately he made arrangements to enter such a clinic, and at the same time he registered for university courses. He stated that this experience was the turning point in his life and that "It was here that I learned to face, to accept, and to believe in the idea that 'Once a stutterer always a stutterer,' but that it is possible to whittle down the problem to inconsequential proportions."

He attributed the improvement in his speech to a modification of the stuttering pattern, a reduction of avoidance, and the development of a realistic attitude toward his problem. He maintained an interest in further self improvement and has continued at intervals to attend stuttering therapy sessions.

As indicated in the previous evaluations, he commented in his autobiography that he has found that whatever he can do to share with, and to help motivate other stutterers, has given greater meaning to his life.

During the years that Victor has been working on his speech and acquiring his advanced education, he has attended several different universities. Much of the therapy he has received for his stuttering has included significant amounts of psychotherapy. This, in turn, seems to have helped him alter his self-concept, which according to the evaluations presented here, is a realistic one which has enabled him to achieve his goal of teaching.

EVALUATION BY THE THERAPIST

Victor has speech which is very good. Frequently the untrained observer might never be aware of his problem. The speech patterns are as well controlled as any I have seen. The tendencies are there, but his excellent control techniques make performance good. He has made quite a good adjustment to his stuttering and readily admits his role of a fluent stutterer. He insists that he must feel free to stutter, if necessary, but even then, it is possible to stutter and still be fluent. This, no doubt, serves to keep anxiety about speech reduced.

Summary and Conclusions

This chapter has endeavored to show the importance of an individual's self-concept in influencing his behavior and personality organization. It has been concerned specifically with the self-concept of stutterers. The thesis has been that a great deal of the therapy administered to stutterers is psychotherapy and in turn successful psychotherapy alters the self-concept of the subject advantageously. The authors hypothesized that psychotherapy was an effective agent in helping the stutterer deveop a more realistic, accurate and mature self-concept.

Rogers has stated that psychotherapy produces sufficient change in the recipient so that the "self" and the "ideal" grow closer together, and therefore the self-concept has changed for the better.

In the process the goals of the subject have been altered. The personality the stutterer would like to project now "has become less perfect, less "adjusted," more realistic, thus becoming a more achievable goal" (13 p. 418). Also the perception he has of others has been changed, and the gap between the client's self-concept and his evaluation of other people is considerably lessened.

Often the person who enters therapy has a picture of himself which is far removed from—or even negatively correlated with—the real self. In general, then, the stutterer seeking help at the speech clinic often sees himself as very unlike the person he really is. Many times his conception of the person he wants to be is also unrealistic. He is apt to be in distress and mal-adjusted. During therapy he becomes more comfortable with himself and moves in the direction of adjustment and integration. He understands himself better and is more apt to alter his goals so they become more true to life. Rogers and his associates concluded from their research that the new self-concept developed during psychotherapy included more of the subject's inner experience, and therefore he was less easily threatened (13).

Raimy (12) found that successful counseling resulted in a change in the client's self-concept, but this shift in self-evaluation did not occur in unsuccessfully counseled clients.

Following is a condensed summary of the evaluations of the subjects discussed in this chapter. It tends to substantiate the hypothesis that therapy helps the stutterer develop a more accurate self-concept.

Subject I - Claude

W-A-Y Technique—Average answer score: 1.7. As indicated previously, the W-A-Y Technique is scored on a 1 to 4 continuum with 1 representing a self-centered personal response and 4 an altruistic social response. Claude's score of less than 2 indicated that he is self-centered and egoistic, being neither objective nor identifying with a group. He is primarily interested in himself and is not concerned with the welfare of society.

Q-Technique adjustment score: 55. As previously stated, a perfect adjustment score on this test would be 74. Claude's score probably reveals a faulty self-concept and a lack of objectivity toward his problem. This score likely indicates an overcompensation on the subject's part. The rationale for this statement was given earlier.

In the Stuttering Behavior Analysis the great discrepancy in Claude's evaluation of his speech and the evaluation given him by the other members of the group supports the conclusion drawn from his Q-adjustment score that his self-concept was not true to life.

Claude's autobiography reconfirmed the unrealistic concept he had of himself as being a normal speaker. Unlike most severe stutterers, he stated that he had never been embarrassed because of his problem. It will be interesting to re-evaluate Claude's self-concept after he has received therapy for several months.

Subject II - Mark

W-A-Y Technique—Average answer score: 2.3. While Mark had not completely identified with the group, he tended toward less personal answers and more general responses.

Q-Technique adjustment score: 41. This slightly above average score appeared to correspond with his observed social behavior. The Stuttering Behavior Analysis Chart confirmed this realistic self-concept Mark had of himself. The subject's autobiography revealed an objective attitude with the realization that his poor speech was a handicap, but the problem could be surmounted. The "man he thought he was" seemed to be in harmony with "the man he was."

Subject III - Victor

W-A-Y Technique—Average answer score: 2.9. The score obtained by Victor supports the findings of Zelen and associates (19) and other research workers (1, 12) that positive feelings increase and negative feelings decrease with successful psychotherapy.

Q-Technique adjustment score: 49. This was in harmony with his social behavior and was felt to be a true assessment of his self-concept.

The Stuttering Behavior Analysis substantiated the findings from the other instruments in that it indicated that Victor's self-concept was realistic. This same realism was shown in the autobiography.

Résumé

The autobiographies of the three subjects proved to be a valuable source of information and provided many interesting clues regarding each subject's self-concept. It was interesting to note that there were other stutterers in the immediate families of two of the three subjects. The other subject, Victor, stated in his autobiography that he had distant relatives who stuttered.

From the foregoing it appears that the evaluations discussed here will permit professional workers to obtain a reasonably accurate picture of the self-concepts of stutterers referred to them. It also appears that therapy administered to relieve stuttering is psychotherapeutic, and this enables individuals to gain a more realistic self-concept.

Today, as in the past, the answer to the age-old problem depicted by the word "nitit" remains hidden. Nevertheless, with all of the different avenues being investigated at the present time, the enigma of "nitit" should, before too long, unmask its mystery.

References

1. Bugental, J. F. T. and Zelen, S. L.: Investigations into the 'self-concept'. I. The W-A-Y technique. *J. Personality 18:* 483-498, 1950.
2. Calzia, G. Panconcelli: *Geschichtszahlen Der Phonetik, 3000 Jahre Phonetik.* Hamburg 11, Hansischer Gildenvealog, 1941.
3. Clark, Ruth M.: Group therapy for young stutterers—panel on the stutterer in our public schools, Leon Lassers, Chairman. *Western Speeches, 15:* 25, 1951.
4. Clark, Ruth Millburn and Fitzpatrick, J. A.: Self-concept in diagnosis and therapy, in *The Psychotherapy of Stuttering.* Dominick A. Barbara, ed. Springfield, Charles C Thomas, 1962.
5. Curtis, W. D.: Agreement between personal descriptions in autobiography and inventory. Unpublished doctoral dissertation, University of Denver, 1960.
6. Dymond, Rosalind F.: Adjustment changes over therapy from self-sorts, in *Psychotherapy and Personality Change.* Rogers and Dymond, eds., Chicago, University of Chicago Press, 1954.
7. Fiedler, F. E. and Wepman, J. M.: An exploratory investigation of the self-concept of stutterers. *J. Speech Hearing Dis. 16:* 110, 1951.

8. Freeman, B. B.: Evaluating W-A-Y technique in relationship to measurement and stability of the self-concept. Unpublished doctoral dissertation, University of Denver, 1956.

9. Goldberg, Alvin: The Q-sort in speech and hearing research. *Asha, 4:* 255, 1962.

10. Johnson, W., Darley, F. C. and Spriesterbach, D. C.: *Diagnostic Methods in Speech Pathology.* New York, Harper and Row, 1963.

11. Parks, W. A.: An exploratory study of self-concept. Unpublished Master of Art Thesis, University of Denver, 1951.

12. Raimy, V. C.: Self reference in counseling interviews. *J. Consult. Psychol., 12:* 153-163, 1948.

13. Rogers, C. R.: An overview of the research and some questions for the future in *Psychotherapy and Personality Change.* Rogers and Dymond, eds., Chicago, University of Chicago Press, 1954.

14. Schilder, P.: *The Image and Appearance of the Human Body.* New York, International Universities Press, 1950.

15. Snygg, D. and Combs, A. W.: *Individual Behavior: A New Frame of Reference for Psychology.* New York, Harper and Brothers, 1949.

16. Speech Foundation of America: *On Stuttering and its Treatment:* Memphis, Tennessee, 1960.

17. Strang, Ruth: *Counseling Techniques in College and Secondary School.* New York, Harper and Brothers, 1949.

18. Watson, R. I. and Mensh, I. N.: The evaluation of the effects of psychotherapy. *J. Psychol., 32:* 259-308, 1951.

19. Zelen, S. L., Shechan, F. G. and Gugental, J. F. T.: Self-perceptions in stuttering. *J. Clin. Psychol., 10:* 70-72, 1954.

8

An Experiment into the Team Approach
To Group Psychotherapy with Stutterers

Dominick A. Barbara, M.D.

Since the beginning of the psychoanalytic movement with Freud, the aims of the psychotherapeutic method have undergone considerable change and development. The main goal was then symptom removal. Today the emphasis is away from symptoms as prime expressions of underlying disturbances and toward the treatment of the total personality. This holistic approach involves focusing not only on the individual's disturbances in relation to others, but also on the nature and importance of intrapsychic tenets. Inherent in its philosophical tenets is the belief that "man can change and go on changing as long as he lives," and that in him there are evolutionary constructive forces which urge him to realize his potentialities. Finally, a comprehensive therapeutic approach must involve not only the early development of the individual, but also the basic conflicting tendencies throughout all phases of his life, with an understanding of both his constructive and destructive (inhibiting) forces. With these pertinent data at hand, therapy may now be directed toward a reorientation of the individual, by making available to him whatever constructive resources are possible toward a healthy growth. The more the individual is helped and directed toward liberating the forces of spontaneous growth, the more awareness, understanding, and a "sense of being" will he have for himself. In short, the ideal in any worthwhile psychotherapeutic approach is the liberation and cultivation of those forces which lead to self-realization.

Stuttering as a speech impediment is a detriment both to the personality and socially. As a symptom, it can be considered, in this context, as an outward expression of anxiety in conflict, secondary to an unhealthy personality development and is manifested specifically and implicitly in speaking where the lines of normal verbalization and communication are disturbed. Finally, the stutterer in his speech difficulty tells us that his lines of communication are broken not only with the world about him, but also in relation to himself. Therefore it is essential that we approach the stutterer as a whole person, suffering from unhealthy relationships and neurotic difficulties which become expressed overtly when he speaks and especially so at the moment of stuttering. Only after we are able to help him find himself and work through his innermost confusion and entanglements, will he find real inner balance and subsequently achieve healthy coordination of his feelings and actions—including that of relaxed and spontaneous speech.

In her excellent book *Neurosis and Human Growth,* Karen Horney[1] clearly writes: "We want to help the patient himself, and with that the possibility of working toward his self-realization. His capacity for good human relations is an essential part of his self-realization, but it also includes his faculty for creative work and that of assuming responsibility for himself. . ."

Briefly, the following are some of the essential aims in therapy:

1) To remove those obstructive forces which are in the path of the patient's motivations for seeking help. People who come into therapy want to be helped because of their stuttering, phobias, headaches, difficulties in speaking or communication, inhibitions in work etc. However, although the above symptoms appear to be sufficient reasons for undergoing treatment and would not require further examination, the essential question to be asked is not "what is being disturbed?", but "who is disturbed?"

2) To help the patient overcome all those needs, drives, or attitudes which obstruct his growth as a whole; so that he can relinquish his illusions about himself and his illusory goals. In so

doing, he can develop realistic self-concepts about himself and the world about him, and thus discover his true potentialities, real feelings, wishes, beliefs and ideals. Only when he faces these issues squarely, can he evolve a solid self-confidence, remove his existing conflicts and ultimately have a chance for real integration.

3) Finally, the road of psychoanalytic therapy, as in the terms of Socrates and Hindu philosophy, is the road to reorientation through self-knowledge: The therapist helps the patient to become aware of the forces operating in him, the extent to which these same forces create anxiety and cause his symptomatology, the nature of his obstructive and constructive attitudes, and in due course, to assist him to combat the former and to mobilize the later. Though the undermining of the obstructive forces and the simultaneous mobilization of the constructive ones, real growth ensues, and the symptoms slowly disappear. However for all of this to be realized, a knowledge of one's self must not remain on the intellecutal level, but must become an emotional experience.

Team Approach to the Therapy of Stuttering

In the recently edited book, *The Psychotherapy of Stuttering,* Villarreal[2] writes:

> The term "team approach" is used with increasing frequency to describe therapeutic programs in which a number of specializations work together co-operatively in a complicated rehabilitation process. What is being recommended here is a team approach for the problems of stuttering, an approach in which the therapy team includes the skills and orientation of a speech therapist and the skills and orientation of a psychotherapist.
>
> It should be pointed out that what is being insisted upon here is not that the union lines between the speech pathologist and the psychotherapist be rigorously preserved, or that penalties be invoked when the one threatens to cross over into the domain of the other. There is nothing inherent in the situation that makes it impossible for a single person to possess and to employ whatever special talents may be peculiar either to the speech pathologist or the psychotherapist. Quite a few individuals think they possess, and a somewhat smaller number can demonstrate by the programs of training they have followed that they do possess, the skills of both speech pathology and psychotherapy. There are persons who are Fellows of the American Speech and

Hearing Association, and either Diplomats of the American Psychological Association or holders of a medical degree with specialization in psychiatry, or both!

What is being said is that persons with this breadth of professional training are rare, and are not ever likely to be numerous, and are certain to be far less numerous than is needed for the treatment of stuttering. It follows, then, that if an adequate program of therapy for stutterers will generally require the special talents both of the speech pathologist and the psychotherapist, most of the practitioners in either field will be inadequately prepared to perform both functions well, and the team approch is called for.

A therapy program along the lines that have been described is approximated, although perhaps not exploited to the fullest possible extent, in a number of programs already in existence. These programs possess all, or most, of the following characteristics:

1) Therapy for the problem of stuttering is viewed as a joint activity of a therapy team that includes a speech pathologist and a clinical psychologist or psychiatrist.

2) The diagnostic examination of the stutterer includes attention to the vocal-mechanism centered aspects, superintended by a speech pathologist, and attention to the emotional health of the stutterer, superinteded by a clinical psychologist. Generally, the stutterer will be administered a battery of such tests as the clinical psychologist has available, particularly projective tests, that are held to be capable of throwing light on the state of emotional health of a person.

3) There will be abundant opportunities for interaction by the two therapies, with consultations at the diagnostic level, joint plannings of therapy activities, and assessment that is broad enough to include evidences of speech fluency and evidences of emotional health as well.

The Therapeutic Approach

A detailed presentation of treatment in stuttering cannot be given in one chapter; only the basic principles and methods of effective treatment are mentioned here. Aside from the preventive and educational procedures of value in all disease entities, treatment in this particular context will be undertaken from a combined psychotherapeutic and speech technique.

The adult stutterer, in contrast to the child stutterer, is consciously aware that he has a speech difficulty and is particularly affected by what others think of him. He develops a keen sensitivity concerning his affliction and is easily affected by criticism and his own particular shortcomings. Treatment in this stage consists primarily of a direct approach. The individual's problems are tackled directly and the aim is toward personality and speech organization.

1) Intake Interviews: The initial interview has many important functions. It can be used for diagnostic means, prognostic or therapeutic purposes, and also as a medium to help the patient prepare for future therapy. In this meeting, we are in a strategic position to get a bird's-eye view of the person who is seeking help. We learn a great deal about him through our first impressions and intuitive feelings. We can also gather pertinent facts about him through our observations of him as he greets us, his manner of approach, his gait, his posture and physical proportions, his smile, his mood, his voice, the color of his eyes, the condition and grooming of his hair, the texture of his skin, the way he wears his clothes. These and many more overt manifestations can be utilized in helping us to understand his personality make-up and the possible attitudes and ways in which he experiences living.

The initial interview is also a basic source of a number of important facts and data the therapist must know about his patient before beginning adequate therapy. Briefly, these include: name, age, sex, marital status, occupation, religion, education, social status, family background, sibling relations, medical history, early childhood, adolescence and adult development, and sexual history. During this first interview the patient also describes his immediate symptoms and complaints. (In addition, a detailed record of all symptoms and complaints, and primarily that of stuttering, is of prime importance.) The therapist should ask for information as to the age at the onset of stuttering, how and where it started, its connection with any traumatic experience or experiences, and when the person first began to associate the first objective and subjective feelings of anxiety with his speech defect. In this same orientation it is important to seek data concerning a specific familial history of stuttering, parental attitudes toward his speaking and toward his speech defect, and, most essential of all, the patient's own feelings and attitudes about his stuttering throughout his remembered development. Finally, for a more complete picture, it is necessary to have some understanding of the patient's present attitudes about his speech impediment, and especially how he experiences it in relation to himself and others. We can now arrive at an initial working premise of the patient's predominant neurotic solutions, the extent to which he uses his stuttering as a neurotic device, and finally some insight into the degree of alienation present.

2) Background Findings: The present investigation was conducted among adult stutterers who were treated in group psychoanalysis at the Karen Horney Clinic. At first, only those individuals who exhibited definite symptoms of stuttering were selected for study. Recently, however, because stutterers as a homogenous group tended to bog each other down and restrict their freedom of expression and spontaneity, a heterogeneous group of stutterers and non-stutterers was chosen. This latter combination proved to be much more effective therapeutically.

The group of stutterers comprised eight men and two women, all unmarried. Five members are in their thirties, four in their twenties, one in his forties. Professional people and students make up the majority. Six are in college or have graduated, two have M.A.'s and are studying for Ph.D.'s. They are predominantly of Jewish descent. One is of Moroccan-Jewish background, one Italian, and one an African Negro. Otherwise, cultural backgrounds are strongly similar.

In the family histories of these patients, the fathers appear generally as distant, cold, and withdrawn. (It is undoubtedly significant that the two fathers who are remembered as warm died when the patients were small children.) One was obviously extremely demanding, harsh, and punitive, and in another case, where an uncle performed the part of proxy parent, it was again noticeable that excessively high standards were set for the child. In still another case, the child was made to feel responsible for the father's having abandoned his education and a better career. Most of these fathers are described as hardworking wage-earners; only one was irresponsible — the "weak and lazy" type. In general, these patients seem to have been much closer to their mothers than their fathers.

In six of the parental marriages, the mother was the dominant figure in the household. Five of the mothers seem to have been very possessive and interfering. Three were obviously overprotective and three excessively demanding. Two were remote because of death or frequent absence from home.

Three of the parental marriages were openly unhappy, with much friction observed by the child. In two of the cases there were temporary or permanent separations.

None of these patients is an only child. Two are the eldest of the siblings and one the eldest of his sex. Only one was the youngest. Five come from families of three, the others from families ranging from two to five children. The information on the relationships to their siblings is sparse, but in several cases the patient recalls sharp antagonism to one or more brother or sister. On the other hand, two of the men make a point of their closeness to their brothers and one of his closeness to his sister, who was in the position of a mother-substitute.

In childhood, eight of these patients recall themselves as having been conforming, shy, withdrawn, and often fearful. (One of these was aggressive in his earliest years, and then changed completely to shy, withdrawn behavior in later childhood.) Of the other two, one was a lively "scrapper," an outstanding athlete who was very severely disciplined for misbehavior, while the last one recalls little of his childhood. His relation to parents seems to have been cold and distant.

Seven of these patients started to stammer in the pre-school period, one when he was six, one when he was eleven, and one in high school. Material on the possible precipitating incident is very scarce. One patient recalled being criticized for poor pronunciation in front of his class. Another associated onset of his symptom with an attack of St. Vitus' Dance. Another believed it began when at the age of four he was sent away from his father to live with his uncle, who was a severe stammerer. (In another case, the father and brothers have a slight stammer.) Another remembers the impact of being ridiculed by other children, while a patient who had long had a mild stammer felt it became a great deal worse at the onset of adolescence. One patient thought that a pertinent factor was his rivalry with his twin brother, who was aggressive socially successful, and a particularly articulate and fluent talker.

In many of these interviews, certain aspects of the patient's backgrounds are not covered. It is possible that if the same question had been asked of all the patients, the figures on certain similarities in family relationships and personalities would be much higher.

The complete observations derived from the intake interviews are summarized in the table on the following pages:

*3) Psychological Testing:**   The psychological tests administered to the patients in the stuttering group were the Wechsler Adult Intelligence Scale, Rorschach's Test, Drawings of the Human Figure, Unpleasant Concept, Three Wishes, and Thematic Apperception Test.

Behavior During Testing: The behavior during testing ranged from the very few who were friendly, cooperative, and enthusiastic to the equally few who were suspicious and frightened. For the most part, the stuttering patient was cooperative, interested, and serious about testing. Most patients started testing with marked stuttering which subsided considerably as they became involved, so that many were free of stuttering during most of the testing.

Intellectual Functioning: The I.Q. range appears to be from 102 to 126, a range from average to superior, indicating the group to be generally of good intellectual endowment. For all patients, there is indication of probably higher endowment than was attained on test scores, but negativism, tensions, some indications of impulsivity and impaired judgment interfered with maximum potential functioning. Although there is this blocking in intellectual functioning, it would appear that, for the most part, the intellectual potential of the stuttering group is not so severely limited as in the general range of patients in the Clinic.

Composite Personality of Stutterer as Seen in Testing: Tests delineate the picture of an isolated, hostile person who relates in a marginal manner inasmuch as he is distant from and suspicious of those around him. In addition to distance from others, there is evidence of hostility directed against his milieu. These feelings appear reactive to unsatisfying relations to the parental figures and frustrations about fundamentally being able to relate to others.

---

*This material originally was compiled and summarized by the late Dr. Marvin Chapman, formerly psychologist at the Karen Horney Clinic.

He appears to be a passive, immature individual who feels inadequate, damaged, frightened, and loaded with hostility. Reactive anger is suppressed and externalized so that he tends to see others as punitive and assaultive. Following is an example of a TAT story:

> "This was a . . . it could be a few things. This gentleman was asleep with this lady. He just got up. He's tired. He's wiping his eyes. Or it . . . he did something to her he does not like. He's ashamed and is holding his eyes. He could have killed or raped her. He confesses and he goes to the cops. This looks like some child or some person, leaning on the bed or sitting on the floor, and crying about something. Now that I look at it, there's a pistol on the floor, so it's probably a grown-up and he or she probably shot someone. Had an argument and is sorry for it now. If he shot someone, maybe he'll confess. Otherwise, he'll shoot himself or he already did."

The thought content here suggests a feeling of fear that hostile forces would be unleashed against him from the environment and a concommitant fear that his own latent aggression projected onto others might erupt. Asked to explain the proverb, "Strike while the iron is hot," he said: "Take advantage of the opportunity without having to trample on other people." In giving a similarity between an ax and a saw, he replied: "Both are used for decapitating and murderous purposes." For such a patient, people are distant, uninterested, and unconcerned about others. Since human relations are fraught with instability and unpredictability, the patient feels it dangerous to get involved with others, particularly on a feeling level. There is considerable difficulty in relating to people who are seen as basically authoritarian and injurious. In the suppression of this anger and hostile feelings, the patient has unfortunately inhibited his drive to assert himself and compete with others. A significant part of the records is concerned with unrealistic distortion of the world, which is seen as extremely dangerous, this encouraging further withdrawal. There is an intense inability to tolerate anxiety and an inability to exercise a degree of personal discipline to confront problems directly and to deal with them. There is, in effect, a subtle withdrawal from the everyday world and interpersonal relationships.

Defenses consist of intellectualizing, perfectionist strivings with

Observations From Intake Interviews

Education	Profession	Father's Personality	Mother's Personality	Siblings	Childhood Behavior	Onset of Stammer	Possible Precipitating Event
1. M.A. working on Ph.D.	Student	Pushing, demanding. Patient brought up by strict uncles.	Divorced by father when patient 3 years. No further contact.	1 older sister, 1 brother 7 years younger.	Athletic a "scrapper," very severely disciplined.	Age 4	Sent away from family to live with stammering uncle.
2. M.A. working on Ph.D.	Student	Cold, disinterested.	Over protective, possessive.	Middle child between 2 sisters.	Early childhood aggressive & hostile. Later shy & withdrawn.	"As long as I can remember."	Unknown
3. B.A.	Market research	Frustrated in job. Patient made to feel responsible.	Possessive, interfering over-close.	1 brother 8 years younger.	Conforming, conscientious.	Third year high school.	Criticized for pronunciation in front of class.
4. H.S.	Student	Rigid, severe, punitive, demanding.	Nervous, fearful, destructive, interfering.	Middle child. Older brother, younger sister.	Shy, withdrawn, lonely.	"As long as I can remember."	
5. H.S.	Office worker	Unreliable, weak, treated with contempt by family.	Sharp-tongued, argumentative, domineering.	1 brother and sister older. 1 sister younger.	Conscientious, fearful, shy. Hostile but dependent relation to mother.	Pre-school	Unknown

		Father	Mother	Siblings	Patient	Onset	Precipitating factor
6. C.S.	College student	Quiet, hard-working, withdrawn.	Outgoing, but dominant, explosive.	2 brothers, younger.	Unclear, some acting out in school. Relation to parents cold.	"As long as I can remember."	Unknown. Father and brother also stammer.
7. H.S. equivalent	Hotel manager	No description. Seems cold, attended to physical needs only.	Same as father.	2 older sisters, 1 younger sister.	Dutiful, obedient, conforming, lonely.	Pre-school	Unknown
8. H.S.	Secretary-bookkeeper	Died when patient was 7 years. "Quiet," good husband and father.	Neurotic, excitable domineering, given to fantasies	Fourth of 5 children.	Shy, timid, sickly.	Age 6	Attack of St. Vitus Dance.
9. College student	Student	Died when patient was 5. Warm, jolly, kind.	Not close, cut off by culture, language, economic circumstances. Demanding.	2 sisters; youngest of 3.	"Good boy," but frightened of dark, nightmares.	Age 11	Ridicule of other children.
10. Twenty-five points short of B.A.	Furniture polisher, musician	Quiet, lonely, withdrawn.	Social, lively, dominant, self-sacrificing.	Fraternal twin, 1 sister, 11 years younger.	"Miserable" because of speech. Close to mother, unhappy about parental conflict.	Pre-school	Unknown, but rivalry with articulate twin probably a factor.

a pervasive depressive mood reflecting disappointment in human relations, confusion in identity with confused sexual aims and an underlying grandiosity and expansiveness to compensate for feelings of weakness and helplessness resulting from the feeling that others do not care about him. All of which is repressed beneath a facade of excessive compliance.

In summary, it was found that: a) The personality of the majority of stutterers studied appeared to be of a schizoid make-up; b) The I.Q. of the group ranged from 102 to 126, indicating a good degree of intellectual endowment; c) The stutterer for the most part is a hypersensitive, tense, anxious, and introverted person. His relationships to himself and to others about him are disturbed. He tends toward intellectualizations, externalizations, and perfectionistic strivings, with a pervasive feeling of underlying hopelessness and resignation, d) finally, his family constellation consists mainly of a dominant, over-protective or perfectionistic, self-sacrificing mother and a father who is for the most part aloof, indifferent, detached, and remains in the background.

4) The Process of Group Psychoanalysis: Once the primary objectives are established and a plan of approach is decided upon by the therapist, more possible and productive therapeutic work can begin. In accordance with the original premises of this paper, especially that of promoting self-realization, it is important early in the therapeutic process to recognize the various resistances and blockages that are keeping neurotic process going and, simultaneously, are interfering with healthy growth. Since we are primarily interested in helping the patient find himself, we must help remove those obstacles which obstruct his growth, interfere with his real self, and cause him to feel alien to himself and to others.

According to Sidney Rose:[3]

> ". . . processes are in operation in group and in individual analysis — namely, spotting neurotic facets of the personality, gradual emergence of such facets into greater awareness, experiencing conflict, experiencing the consequences of neurotic integrating patterns—i.e., their destructiveness to one's best self-interest, the awareness of externalizations, and the re-internalizing of externalized aspects of the self—and the activating of the latent growth potentials in each one."

The group situation is of considerable importance to stutterers because it creates a situation in which the stutterer is brought face to face with himself and to experience himself as he really is, and how he may appear to the other members of the group. It can become, as Benjamin Becker[4] puts it:

> "a broader experience of self-awareness and awareness of others through a valuable and increasingly freer contact with people. The constructive potentials, the essentially unconscious forces of strength and health, which are buried and imprisoned by the neurotic character structure of each patient, are encouraged to emerge in this very human group process."

The group therapy situation is also important in that it helps the stutterer to see that others, especially those who may be non-stutterers, have similar difficulties, conflicts, struggles — that he is not alone in his troubled situation. This important subjective feeling of being "in the same boat with others" ultimately adds to his own self-growth. And, in the case of stutterers, it gives them the valuable experience of seeing other people stutter and of learning from their difficulties.

In the group situation, in contradistinction to individual therapy, the stutterer is more willing to accept his own limitations and discrepancies when he realizes that he shares them with others. It also helps him to move closer to those others in the group and, in general, improve his relations with others.

The stutterer, who is usually beset by self-criticism, finds in the group situation a means of expressing himself as freely as possible without inhibition or censorship. In so doing, he can gain valuable insight into many of his defenses, prejudices, illusions, blind spots, and various aspects of his speech difficulty. The group situation can now be used as a proving ground for testing the validity and reliability of inner feelings and constructive changes in himself.

Finally, the group milieu gives the therapist a "real-life" situation in which to observe his patient with his various attitudes, feelings, and beliefs, especially as these factors operate in relation to others. Material of this sort is of importance for discussion and elaboration in those instances where the stutterer may be simultaneously undergoing individual treatment.

5) Working Directly with Resistances in the Stutterer:
Undermining the Demosthenes Complex: One of the more destructive and self-perpetuating forces in neurosis is that of self-
idealization. The neurotic's illusory image of himself, with its accompanying pride values, has to be undermined in order for him to
have a chance to feel himself and evaluate his more real and basic
potentialities.

The stutterer, though basically similar in structure to other
neurotics, may be said nevertheless to present characteristic differences in his orientation toward life. Because of his particular
make-up, his early interpersonal relations, and his accentuation on
anxiety and fears in the speaking situation, there is created in him
an idealized image of his own particular need to compensate for
his own sense of inadequacy in this area. I refer to this process of
self-glorification in stuttering as the Demosthenes Complex.

In the case of the person who stutters, his exaggerated sense of
self-importance, his vanity and egocentricity, interfere with his
having a real sense of self-confidence. This, along with his illusions
of himself as the "perfect orator" in the speaking situation has to be
undermined in order for him to make fewer imaginary claims upon
himself and others, leading ultimately to a feeling of more solid
inner strength.

B. Bohdan Wassell[5], in his book on group psychoanalysis, writes
that the unique advantage of the group in therapy is the uncov-
ering of "universal illusions," the oscillating feelings of pride and
self-contempt, the basic anxiety common to all neurotics. Each one
learns that the others are as frightened and anxious as he is. Each
one asks the same questions as to his identity, how he fits in, how
he compares with others, what others value, and so forth. In the
process of working together, the group develops a spirit that is an
important background of feeling, akin to rapport in individual
analysis and almost as difficult to define and demonstrate as the
soul. This group spirit develops out of feelings of mutual respect
and affection for each other. Also, in group therapy, the actual
disillusionment process — which can be of a very painful nature in
individual therapy — is better tolerated by the patient because of
this same spirit of group acceptance and support.

Difficulties in Beginning Therapy: A major problem in the

treatment of stuttering is how to encourage the stutterer to stay in and continue with the course of treatment. This, of course, involves first of all an evaluation of the real incentives in the individual patient and what his expectations will be, once he consents to start therapy.

Doubts and feelings of doom have become fixed in the minds of many stutterers who have gone from clinic to clinic, from specialist to specialist, or have been subjected to so-called "miraculous cures." When these unfortunates are initially interviewed for what they may feel is another futile attempt, they often are skeptical and cautious. They have little real incentive to receive help in the solution of their problems and a difficult area of resistance is set up. Many times, in these instances, the therapist must give a great deal of himself initially by way of encouragement.

Group therapy is most beneficial in ameliorating the stutterers' pessimism about themselves. To quote from a recent article by Benjamin Becker:[6] "It requires courage for the patient to move forward in the psychoanalytic process. It is the courage of the pioneer, who is moving into unexplored territory fraught with unknown dangers with which he must cope using new and untried weapons. Although growth and change are normal phenomena of human living, transition is not easy at any stage of a person's development and more difficult if there are neurotic impediments. Patients are often gripped by pessimism about their eventual growth. Their faith in themselves and in the therapeutic process sometimes wanes. In the group, people draw courage from the constructive efforts of the others as a whole. At times group insecurity, uneasiness, and pessimism may come through. But with repeated positive experiences, patients relate to one another with greater confidence."

To help remove those resistances which are perpetuated by the stutterer's disturbed productivity and intellectualizations: Besides the stutterer's hesitations when speaking, he presents similar inhibitions and blocks in the quality of his productions. The stutterer is known to block with his whole organism — his feelings, attitudes, beliefs, and actions.

The stutterer thinks highly of "wisdom" and "intellect." His thinking is usually in terms of absolutes. His responses are purely on an intellectual level. His own inner fear of feelings forces him to seek logical and clean-cut answers to his problems. Seeking his conflicts at a distance, he tries to compartmentalize and rationalize his shortcomings and opposing tendencies.

The group therapeutic process is very valuable as a constructively oriented setting wherein people can congregate and experience the quality of their relations with others. At the beginning, each stutterer in a group situation may set himself apart as an isolated and fortified entity of his own. He will use his intellect to ward off any intimate contact with others in the group milieu, and resort to other defensive tactics, so his protective armor will not be penetrated. However, as the members of the group get to know each other, they find areas of similarity and dissimilarity amongst them selves, develop further understanding of the meaning of the process they are engaged in, and finally draw more closely together. They feel freer to express both their thoughts and emotions, envision each other as human beings, and as a result there is less fear, not only of what the others might think or say, but also of their own anxieties and vulnerabilities.

The actual stuttering symptom is one of the major blockages in productivity. The therapist struggling to remove the symptom itself and not working with the total character structure is easily caught in a tangle of intellectual discussions on the presupposed cause-and-effect correlations of stuttering.

In the group process, it is essential not to deal specifically with the stuttering manifestation, but to understand what the stutterer is trying to express when he speaks, and especially at the time he stutters. The therapist must intercept and decode the messages the stutterer sends by the way he presents himself in speaking, his hidden meanings, feeling tones, anxieties, inhibitions, hesitations, and especially his own word jargon.

In the group situation, stutterers tend to externalize their difficulties and conflicts onto each other. For the most part, the stutterer feels apart and different from others in his society. He may feel that although others also have difficulties in life, they can cope with them and live more easily with their problems. He feels more permanently crippled than others because of the fact that he cannot hide or conceal his speech difficulty. He may rationalize to the effect that persons with migraine headaches, hard-of-hearing, asthma, and ulcers suffer, but they can still keep their troubles to themselves and go on living, while he, unable to speak fluently, has the added burden of social criticism and judgment. The stutterer makes tenacious claims that the world should provide him special services and privileges and entitle him to a "position in life," "a job suitable to his speech incapacity," "a society which will make allowances for his stuttering," yet at the same time not make it too obvious that he is afflicted. These latter externalizations and claims need special attention in the group therapeutic situation and become more easily worked through in a heterogenous group than in an "all-stutterer" group, because of the possibility for comparison and realistic evaluation.

The average speaker usually experiences his speech as his own and as originating from within himself. He feels a choice of his own words or group of words, though there may be some indecision as to word pronunciation. Once he makes his decision and voluntarily chooses his words, he will have little difficulty in consummating the speaking itself. The person who tends to stutter, however, generally experiences his speech as alien to himself and as coming from somewhere outside of himself. His dilemma in speaking is experienced not so much in terms of "what to say" but "how to say it," with all of its explicit and implicit perfectionistic claims. In this sense, the group situation offers the stutterer a unique opportunity to hear himself as he speaks to compare his speaking and its associated attitudes with the other members of the group, and, finally, to act against his symptom in the specific situation that usually provokes it. And, most important of all, in a heterogenous group setting, he learns to understand and feel that he is not so different from non-stutterers, and that most differences are soon minimized as people get to know each other and visualize their difficulties through spontaneous group interaction.

To help alleviate disturbances in the therapist-patient relationship: The transference relationships among the participants in the group and between patients and therapist constitute one of the important aspects of the therapeutic process. Blockages in the course of therapy find their expression chiefly in these transference relationships.

In the specific treatment of stuttering, the stutterer's use of magical claims creates a formidable obstructing force in the therapeutic relationship. He further externalizes his feelings of magic onto the therapist and to the other members of the group, endowing them with qualities that are unrealistic and thus impossible to attain. The therapist becomes unique, is imagined as a magician who can and should easily and effortlessly rid him of his dilemma. At those times when he feels that his therapist or those of the group see through his maneuvers, the stutterer may use his affliction, with all of its appeals, distractions, and rituals, in a desperate drive to restore his weakening defenses. Through all of this, the therapist's real self comes through if shown to advantage, and his closeness to himself enables him to develop better relatedness with his group. The stutterer, despite his show of reluctance, secretly and truly wishes his therapist to be balanced, firm, and consistent for the most part. Only in this way will the therapist ultimately receive the stutterer's real respect and regard, and be able to give him a true sense of security.

To relieve the stutterer of his fears regarding any disturbance to his status quo: The stutterer lives in constant dread of having his protective structures invaded or removed, with the accompanying terror of crumbling and psychically going to pieces. His tolerance for struggle is at a low ebb and this can prove to be a most threatening block in the group situation. He fears open discussion or any direct criticism of himself, for he cannot face his conflicts squarely or bear their related anxiety.

The stutterer fears any open display of emotions and protects himself by hiding behind a facade of intellectualizations, evasions and rationalizations. Should these defenses fail in turn, he may resort to stuttering, or retreat by pleading helplessness and having abused feelings. Or, further, he may avoid the conflict entirely by resigning himself to a state of pseudo-unity. In so doing, he feels he is able to save face in at least part of the struggle.

In this particular area of blockage, the group plays a most important role. The interrelatedness of the group milieu helps the stutterer to begin to see himself less as "just a stutterer" and more as a human being, despite his stuttering. He is helped to feel more hopeful and on firmer ground and, conversely, less resigned and frustrated. His anxieties and the threat to his "loftly position" becomes lessened; he becomes able to take a stand in relation to his conflicts and to have the courage not only to face himself as he really is but also to change.

The Role of the Speech Therapist

If speech therapy is to continue its development and serve the needs of the individual, the therapist, according to Pellman[7], "must consider how it is related to the broader areas of the social sciences. This will serve to eliminate a mechanical approach which, at one time, seemed to make the speech therapist merely some type of mechanic making motor adjustments. Today's speech therapist realizes that when some aspect of remedial speech work is sought, what is being really asked of him is help in fields intimately connected with personality and human development."

In our particular project at the Karen Horney Clinic, a dynamically oriented certified speech therapist, worked in separate meetings with the stutterers in the groups; and, many times attended the actual group sessions, where he participated freely in group discussions. His main role was to listen and gather as much information as he could regarding what was communicated in the group interaction. Simultaneously, there was a constant communication between the psychotherapist and the speech therapist. Pertinent information on what was going on which related to the work of each other was exchanged, and reactions of both therapist were evaluated intermittently.

Speech therapy was presented not as an isolated mechanistic phenomenon, but as a dynamic social function. Productive communicative speech was encouraged, in that it fostered alive, healthy conversational patterns and tended to create movement in the speaker. Little emphasis was placed on *"what was being said,"* but on *"how is was expressed," "what feelings were revealed"* and finally, *"what effect did it produce on the speaker."* Although muscular retraining techniques were used to break down old disturbed speech habits; the speech therapist essentially attempted to connect this physiological impairment with those attitudes which primarily hampered it with contradictary mental sets. In so doing, the therapist not only introduced healthy precepts of real life situations, but simultaneously attempted to ameliorate the existing speech difficulty by introducing newer attitudes which could foster communication.

Although the stutterer can be helped by the psychotherapist with his emotional difficulties as they effect his inter-personal relationships and his attitude toward speech itself; I agree with Bleumel, that simultaneous and sustained efforts at reorganizing basic speech will ultimately prove to give the most curative results.

To quote from Bleumel:[8]

It is only in recent years that the distinction between primary and secondary stammering has been generally understood. Yet the distinction is simple, and it is one that the stammerer, in his efforts at self-help, must keep clearly in mind. The primary disorder is a blocking or muting of the mind which prevents the speaker from thinking the words clearly and saying them clearly. The secondary component is the speaker's reaction to his dilemma and his attempt to battle with it. The speaker must contend with these two conponents in different ways. He must recognize the fact that the secondary speech struggle is not the real difficulty. The panic, the breath-holding, the contortion, the forcing, the aversion and avoidance, the use of starters and wedges and synonyms and circumlocutions are all phases of reaction and they are not part of the primary stammering. When these reactions are recognized as secondary symptoms, they can gradually be minimized and controlled; and the stammerer is then in a better position to contend with the primary speech disorder.

The primary disturbance is the momentary blocking which effaces the mental words from the mind and leaves the speaker mute and confused. The speaker's logical recourse in this situation is to attempt to compose himself and think the words so that he can now say them—clearly and without effort. The illogical recourse is to struggle with the mouth muscles and the breathing muscles and to complicate the picture with a futile struggle reaction. This struggle must be reduced, so that the stammerer is free to deal with his primary disturbance of muting in his inward speech. In this thinking-therapy the speaker looks for fluency just above the ears and not just above the chin. The mind broadcasts to the mouth, and the mouth gives a faithful reproduction of the verbal thinking. It gives the language that is thought, together with the inflection, the articulation, the degree of loudness, and other speech qualities that originate in the mind. There is a parallel in the matter of singing. One must think in tune in order to sing in tune; and if one is off key in singing, it is because one is off key in one's musical thinking. In speech correction one ignores the mouth, and centers the full attention on the mind. If the mental speech is clear and concise, the oral speech will be in similar pattern and the stammering will subside.

There is another area in which the stammerer can strive for fluency; he can seek to improve the general quality of his speech quite apart from the matter of stammering. As already mentioned, facility in speech varies with different people. One man is fluent enough to become a radio commentator; another can scarcely express himself in a fully completed sentence. Thus we see different skills in speaking just as we encounter different skills in singing; and in the case of the stammerer we find a speaker with a rather low level of verbal achievement. Quite apart from the impediment, the stammerer appears to be a non-skilled speaker; he is non-fluent; he carries a speech deficit, as it were. It was probably this non-organization of basic speech that permitted the speech function to become disorganized in early life. But the impediment being established, the frustration continued, and the speech never became organized into a pattern of normal fluency. It is true that the occasional stammerer has occasional fluency, but the fact that this fluency can be shattered by haste or emotion or stress suggests that the function of speech was never organized with any degree of security.

And here lies the stammerer's opportunity—to organize his speech even at a belated period. The procedure is to find occasion to talk in situations that offer relative fluency. This may mean talking or reading alone, reading with a partner or a study group, speaking with records or tape recordings, echoing the speech of a radio or television commentator; in fact, availing oneself of all possible opportunity of hearing and feeling one's speech in un-obstructed fluency. With the basic speech function thus improved, the stammerer is in a good position to monitor his verbal thinking in normal speech situations. He can now broadcast from the mind to the mouth with heightened self-confidence and with considerable fluency.

Conclusion

In the final analysis, the group situation gives the stutterer what he most surely needs — a sense of belonging, an atmosphere of union and unity, a feeling of respect with others, a spirit of group acceptance and support, and finally a controlled environment where he is able to act out his symptom in the specific situation that he feels ordinarily provokes it.

As the stutterer slowly finds himself progressing toward self-realization, he will tend to discard his neurosis and all that it implies, including stuttering.

Whether group analysis in itself is of ultimate benefit to the problem of stuttering, or whether its greatest value may be to complement individual analysis, needs further research and study.

Bibliography

1. Horney, Karen: *Neurosis and Human Growth*. New York, W. W. Norton, 1950.
2. Villarreal, Jesse: The role of the speech pathologist in psychotherapy, in Barbara, D. A., ed.: *The Psychotherapy of Stuttering*. 1962.
3. Rose, Sidney: Group psychoanalysis. *Am. J. Psychoan., XVIII*:-1:69, 1958.
4. Becker, Benjamin J.: Relatedness and alienation in group psychoanalysis. *Am. J. Psychoan., XVIII*:2:150, 1958.
5. Wassell, B. Bohdan: *Group Psychoanalysis*. New York, Philosophical Library, 1959.
6. *Cf.* 4, above: page 152.
7. Pellman, Charles: The relationship between speech therapy and psychotherapy, in Barbara, D. A., ed.: *The Psychotherapy of Stuttering*. 1962.
8. Bleumel, C. S.: Organization of speech as basic therapy, in Barbara D. A., ed.: *The Psychotherapy of Stuttering*. 1962.
9. Barbara, Dominick A.: Communication in stuttering. *Dis. Nerv. Syst.* 9:47:1, 1958.
10. Barbara, Dominick A.: Working with stuttering problem. *J. Nerv. Ment. Dis., 125*:2:329, 1957.
11. Barbara, Dominick A.: *The Psychotherapy of Stuttering*. Charles C Thomas, Springfield, Illinois, 1962.

INDEX